CORONAVIRUS:

(Covid-19)
Tips for Protecting You & Your
Family to Achieve Optimum Health

DR. BRADLEY SHAPERO, D.C.

Library of Congress Cataloging-in-Publication Data
Shapero, Bradley, D.C.
Coronavirus: (Covid-19)
Tips for Protecting You & Your Family to Achieve Optimum Health

Published by Pluma Omnia Vincit, San Clemente, CA

Library of Congress Control Number: 2020913604

Print ISBN: 978-1-7354396-0-0
Digital ISBN: 978-1-7354396-1-7

Cover Design: Lauren Card
Interior Design: Tamara Cribley
Back cover photograph: John J Kallal IV

1. Self-help. 2. Heath. 3. Personal Growth.

PRAISE FOR THE BOOK
CORONAVIRUS

"You will experience an honest and sincere guide which gives you a real picture of the solution, you can feel good that you now have answers to safeguard you and your family."

Dr. Gary Fieber, D.C.

"Like Dr. Shapero, I have been devoted to the practice of healing. While my profession focused on the mind, Dr. Shapero focused on healing the body. In his book on the coronavirus, he draws upon countless years as a chiropractor to offer practical tips to protect you and your family during these turbulent times. Inform yourself and read this book!"

Leonard Szymczak, author of **The Roadmap Home: Your GPS to Inner Peace**

"Dr. Shapero has been an endless source of support for my daughter and myself over the years. His knowledge and selflessness are a true gift. I am beyond grateful. I gained not only an exceptional doctor, but a friend. Thank you for being you."

Britany Doyle, mom, health rights advocate

"I have found a treasure in knowing Dr. Bradley Shapero. I have been in the San Clemente/Dana Point area for 4 years and am thankful to have found him in my search for a chiropractor/ wellness physician. I am a registered nurse and believe in the power of the body's ability to heal itself given the right

support. Dr. Shapero has a vast depth of knowledge of which I believe I have only scratched the surface. Over the years he has shared valuable and practical information concerning nutrition and lifestyle that has been helpful in living a life without fear of disease. My family and I are thankful to know him, be cared for by him, and to glean from his wisdom for a healthier life."

Susan Taylor RN

"Armed with a vast amount of knowledge and enthusiasm for healing, Dr Shapero is impacting people's lives for the better every day. Dr. Brad has a tremendous understanding of the body and knows how to maximize an individual's personal performance. Being involved in Martial Arts for over 35 years, I now refer my martial arts students, of all ages, exclusively to Dr Brad, because I know that they are literally in good hands."

Paul Benavidez, 7th Degree Master Instructor, Zen Dojos Martial Arts Academy

We live in unpredictable times. Some have said we can certainly tell the character of a person by how he or she handles things at a time of crisis.

I dedicate this to those who, despite the challenge, wake up every morning excited to make a difference in a world of chaos and unrest. To all those warriors of health, who continue to go into battle, fighting the good fight despite the odds they may face. To my father Dr. Harris J. Shapero, M.D. z"l (zikhrono livrakha, meaning "May his memory be a blessing") who through his guidance and example showed me how to rise up against the odds, enjoy life while helping others.

TABLE OF CONTENTS

FORWARD

I want to thank Dr. Shapero for his dedication to educate you on an especially important subject. The author has committed his career to helping thousands of patients achieve a healthier and a more stress-free life.

By reading this book, you will experience an honest and sincere guide which gives you a real picture of the solution for you and your family and friends.

Be well and enjoy the fact that you have an answer.

Gary Fieber, D.C., Chiropractor, Consultant

INTRODUCTION

Our world is a fascinating matrix of seemingly organized chaos. As a wellness doctor and chiropractor, I have been serving the community for nearly 30 years. In that time I have found that illness comes about when the threshold of tolerance is overwhelmed. All stress can be compartmentalized into three categories, mental/emotional, physical, and biochemical (which includes both ones nutritional and toxic load status). The world we live in has numerous pathogens such as bacteria, viruses, parasites, molds, and fungi. We also must deal with heavy metals, chemicals and various toxins. How your body deals with each of these considering your individual threshold will indicate your resilience level.

The best way to get or stay healthy is to fortify your castle, which is your body. Maximizing the function and strength of your immune system is the best opportunity to minimize or avoid getting sick. Toxins and pathogens including the coronavirus and in this case the SARS-CoV-2 also have a weakness. SARS-CoV-2 is the official name of the virus by the World Health Organization. The actual name of the disease is called Covid-19. By using common sense and innovative science we can exploit the weaknesses of these invaders while we boost your immune function and lower your stress level.

The fact that the World Health organization has officially classified this as a pandemic should not keep us from our agenda of staying healthy and helping others to do the same. Despite the gloom and doom propagated by the media, solutions are available. Fear will not solve this situation; only consistent swift and smart action will help you through. Inside this book you will learn how to help your body deal with abnormal stress.

It is important to keep in mind that the symptoms of Covid-19 vary greatly from person to person. Symptoms range from very mild achiness, to fever of various degrees, cough and shortness of breath. Some have shown gastrointestinal changes as well. It is also important to note that the vast majority of the individuals who contract the coronavirus recover and are doing great. Those who have had a worse outcome had compromising factors, as well as other disease processes that affected the ability of their immune system to operate effectively. Their bodies became overwhelmed. However, this is a very small percentage of the cases reported. For the average individual the odds are very much in your favor.

Often, life becomes very uncomfortable in the moments preceding great change. Yet, problems become opportunities to think big, learn more, and grow wiser.

Over the years I have helped thousands of moms, dads, children, animals, and individuals just like you. You are about to embark on a fabulous journey. In the pages ahead you will find information to help you understand what Covid-19 is and how to deal with it, as well as reducing stress, improving your immune system, and preparing for this and other situations in the future. You will find tools, tips and strategies you can use to help you stay healthy and minimize your risk.

May this situation with the coronavirus allow us as a community, nation, and world to rethink how we approach the invisible invaders in our world in a way that optimizes health.

- May the information in this book shine light into unseen dark corners and help you grow.
- May it help you assist others as well as give you strength in knowledge to take action.
- May you be healthy and change for the better.

Blessings, Dr. Bradley Shapero, D.C., Wellness Doctor / Chiropractor

CHAPTER ONE

THE OTHER SIDE OF PANIC: UNDERSTAND THE PROBLEM

*Panic causes tunnel vision. Calm acceptance
of danger allows us to more easily assess the
situation and see the options.*

— Simon Sinek

The silence was deafening as I read the text from Ashley. Late in December 2019, I had dinner with her and her relatives visiting from China. Ashley was both excited and apprehensive as she shared about her recent completion of documents pertaining to her citizenship to the US. She, her husband, and newborn baby were heading back to China for a few weeks with her family for the New Year Celebration. The year of the rat.

The text felt surreal, like a movie, although, this movie continued to play with no mute or stop option.

Hi, I am so sorry to have to share this with you.

As you know we landed in Wuhan yesterday. We are okay for now, but my cousin who you met developed a cough on the flight back.

When we landed, he was immediately detained and quarantined for some outbreak which seems to be a disease that has been kept secret from the people until recently, supposedly not to cause a panic. The bad news is that we may have been exposed and infected, including you.

I wasn't sure what this text was all about, but the deep ache in the pit of my stomach could not be calmed. I began to do what most friends would do. I checked the media sources to find out what I could about this mystery disease. As I began my research, I had two questions. How virulent was this thing I was exposed to? What were my risks? Consumed with research, I read for several hours. The more I uncovered, the more I realized that this situation had many faces: the face that China wanted the world to see, the face that was painted by alarmists in the media, and the face of the medical community attempting to walk the line of discovery without overly alarming the public. There was also the face of truth.

Like the old cliché about Vegas, what happened in Wuhan, China was attempting to keep in Wuhan. The rest of the world, however, had a much different take on the situation. I texted Ashley back. *"I am sure glad you let us know. Thank you, I am glad you are alright. Please let us know if something changes or you find out something new about all this. I am going to do some research and I'll let you know what I uncover. Stay Well."*

While I tried to be positive, the last line of her text kept repeating in my mind. *The bad news is that we may have been exposed and infected, including you.*

It was apparent to me the next two weeks would keep us on alert for any change in how we felt. Ashley on the other hand, was quite concerned. She and her family were on self quarantine and were frantically attempting to get her flight changed so she could come home before the proposed travel ban was in place. Meanwhile, not thinking it would be a problem until now, she and her husband were quite aware that his citizenship was not yet complete. It took several calls to the US embassy and lots of prayers to finally get Ashley and her baby on a flight back to the US. After which, she self quarantined for another fourteen days. Her husband was not allowed to leave the country and spent another six weeks in China before he was cleared to travel back to the US and reunite with his wife and baby girl.

Fortunately, I too had not had any symptoms for over a month, well beyond the incubation period. However, my thirst to find out more about what was happening grew stronger.

My search results quickly revealed that the outbreak was a new strain of Coronavirus. The official name of the virus given on February 11, 2020 by the World Health Organization is SARS-CoV-2. The name of the disease is called Covid-19. The virus was initially identified as a new strain of Coronavirus. Researchers were calling it 2019 Novel Coronavirus or #2019nCoV as it was discovered in 2019. I recalled that Coronavirus gathered much recognition in the media with the outbreak of SARS-CoV 2002 and MERS-CoV 2012.

The Coronavirus initially entered the scene in 1965 when Tyrrell and Bynoe discovered they could passage, that is transfer from one tissue or species to another, a virus known as B814. This virus was found in the embryonic tracheal organ cultures obtained from the respiratory tract of an adult with a common cold. The presence of an infectious agent was demonstrated by inoculating[1] the medium from these cultures intranasally in human volunteers; colds were produced in a significant proportion of subjects, but Tyrrell and Bynoe were unable to grow the agent in tissue culture at that time. (Kahn & McIntosh, 2005)

The Coronavirus got its name because under a microscope it resembled an infectious bronchitis virus found in chickens, a spherical shaped particle with club shaped projections on the surface, which gives it a crown like appearance. See Figure 1

This new group of viruses was named coronavirus (corona denoting the crown-like appearance of the surface projections) and was later officially accepted as a new genus of viruses. See Appendix A for more details on this virus. It is a type of airborne pathogen which in this case must be carried on a particle due to its

---

1 To communicate a disease by transferring its virus. In other words obtaining the virus from cultures growing the virus and putting them into the new host.

size, such as a droplet from sneezing or coughing. This is too large to float around in the air.

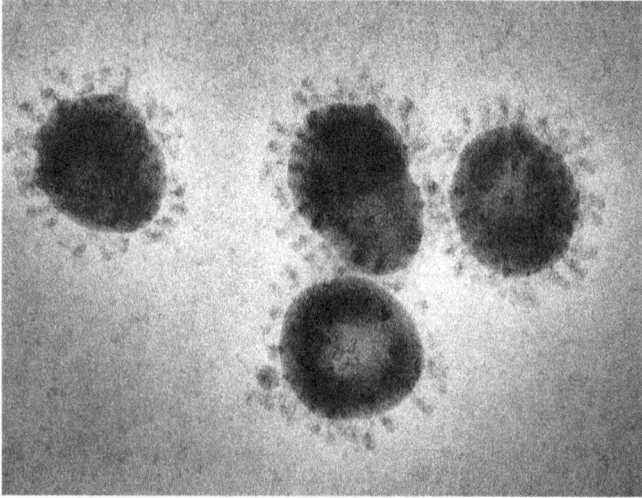

FIGURE 1 Coronavirus.

As is typical with infections, the symptoms do not show up for a period of time after exposure. The amount of delay indicates how quickly it can spread. In the case of CoVid-19, you may not see symptoms for as long as 20 days or more. The estimated delay of infection varies; however, typically the symptoms take anywhere from 2 to 14 days and 4 to 6 days is fairly common.

The reported symptoms range from not being aware you have it to sever multisystem involvement and death. The majority of the cases, over 80%, fall into the mild symptom category. (Coronavirus disease 2019 (COVID-19), 2020) Some people have high fever, loss of taste and smell, along with labored breathing. A small percentage of the population has severe fatigue, fever, shortness of breath, labor of breathing as well as multisystem compromise. As more is uncovered about the reactions people are having, the types of symptoms are evolving to also include skin rashes such as hives, painful swellings on the toes and feet, morbilliform or measles type rash, mottled vascular rashes, vesicle type rash similar to pox, and petechial eruption. In a small percentage of the cases it can even result in death. The initial symptoms most commonly experienced are the following:

- Fever

- Sore Throat

- Dry Cough

- Fatigue (often associated with general malaise or difficulty breathing)

- Shortness of breath

Other symptoms can include:

- Aches

- Vomiting / Diarrhea

- If any of the following symptoms are present immediate medical attention is recommended:

- Ongoing chest pain or pressure

- New confusion

- Difficulty waking up

- Bluish lips or face

Most people have been infected and recovered from infections by one or more different kinds of coronaviruses. The common cold can sometimes be caused by one of four different human coronaviruses, which causes 15 to 30% of common colds. Most colds are caused by rhinoviruses. However, the relatively harmless cold viruses are very different from the novel coronavirus now spreading around the world.

Those at increased risk include the elderly, and those with chronic medical conditions, including diabetes, heart disease, respiratory problems, and weakened or otherwise compromised immune systems.

Now we can move forward to how the Novel Coronavirus came onto the scene. As the name implies it is "novel" which means "of a kind not seen before." We are in a remarkable time in history. Information moves faster than ever, and the volume of data grows far greater every day than we could ever process in one person's lifetime. This is a great opportunity and also a great responsibility for reporting the news and how the discovery of new information is used and disseminated.

Admittedly, it can be challenging to get to the basic truth of some things because of the layers of information. There is the sheer volume of information as well as vested interests in some cases. This creates layers of truth, as well as intentional cover ups which circulate around and take time and energy to uncover. I have made every attempt to sort through this information and will at times share opposing viewpoints so that you can make your own determination and draw your own conclusions.

I have written this book simply to present my findings. The personal stories, in stark contrast to the rest of the book, contain alterations and many names have been changed to make the story more meaningful and relative to the topic. I have cited other sources to make sure the information is accurate. My main focus is to highlight what you can do to protect yourself and those you care about during this outbreak and how to prepare for other outbreaks that may occur. The likelihood that we will see even more lethal pathogens in the future is high, which means it is important to prepare your immune system now for what could present in the future.

You can safeguard your family by getting physically and mentally prepared for a global outbreak or crisis. A crisis can come about in many forms. Fear and panic may arise due to a pathogen which is unknown to the general public. Civil unrest from some social or political disturbance which we have seen can rapidly gain momentum. When this happens we see demonstrations, riots, and other events that destabilize the social, economic, and civil structures we live with today.

As I present this information, I will include various sources which may or may not have been withheld. Outside the shocking conspiracy theory motives, let's keep in mind that there are a multitude of reasons information is withheld in situations like this, as well as some of the very simple reasons. Ask yourself some of these questions:

- Do we have all the facts?

- Did someone make a mistake and unknowingly or carelessly break protocol?

- Was there a monetary motive?

- Do we want to avoid a panic?

- Is there another unknown agenda?

Many answers fall into the realm of reason and are not necessarily malicious. Use your own moral compass to determine if it was dealt with correctly, or not. Appendix B has more history of information about the possible origination of this virus.

Seidel, J. (Jan 29, 2020) Mystery lab next to coronavirus epicenter: News.com.au.

CHAPTER TWO

INFORM YOURSELF: TRUTH AND FAKE NEWS

Whenever the people are well-informed, they can be trusted with their own government.

— Thomas Jefferson

Early in January as I researched the Covid-19 outbreak, a friend, Barbara, contacted me asking for help regarding what she thought was a viral infection. She told me that she had just arrived back from a trip to Italy and seemed fine. Several days later, Barbara did not have enough energy to get out of bed, her breathing was heavy, and oddly enough her sense of smell was impaired. I rapidly put things together and realized Barbara had Covid19. The virus had now crossed the continent. Luckily, due to her symptoms she had been self isolated since she returned. I suspected that those who were in contact with Barbara would soon experience some form of this infection.

She was fortunate that she was better after about day eight of symptoms. However, the more research I came across, the more lines between the truth and fake news were beginning to blur. Separating fact from fiction was becoming more challenging, and even the scientific communities were in debate over the apparent origin.

A look at genomic coding gives us clues to the origin of this novel virus. Here again we move into a highly controversial area. This seems to be an ever changing picture. Somewhat like attempting to grab onto smoke. I have read through dozens of scientific papers on this, and even here the story seems to be changing.

There were claims that this may have been "man-made" and yet some assert that it is a nature made virus. One such claim was reported by Lyons-Weiler for IPAK who made reference to a research paper posted on bioRxiv.org entitled "Uncanny similarity of unique inserts in the 2019-nCoV spike protein to HIV-1 gp120 and Gag" which has subsequently been pulled from the site for further review.

To add to the already wild stories circulating, Federal Agents arrested Dr. Charles Lieber, chair of the Harvard University's Department of Chemistry and Chemical Biology. Lieber was charged with lying to the Department of Defense about secret monthly payments of $50,000.00 paid by China and receipt of millions more to help set up a chemical/biological "Research" laboratory in China. Subsequently, the FBI arrested two Chinese "Students" working as research assistants, one of whom was actually a lieutenant in the Chinese Army, the other captured at Logan Airport as he tried to catch a flight to China smuggling 21 vials of "Sensitive Biological Samples" according to the FBI. (Chastain, 2020)

The research lab this Harvard professor had helped set up was located at the Wuhan University of Technology. Wuhan China is ground zero to the potentially global pandemic known as the 2019-nCoV or Novel Coronavirus which is both spreading rapidly and killing people. As you can imagine this hit the news like wildfire. I must admit this certainly raised some questions. For now here is what I know.

Dr. Charles Lieber, 60, Chair of the Department of Chemistry and Chemical Biology at Harvard University, was arrested and charged by criminal complaint with one count of making a materially false, fictitious, and fraudulent statement. Lieber appeared before Magistrate Judge Marianne B. Bowler in federal court in Boston, Massachusetts.

Yanqing Ye, 29, a Chinese national, was charged in an indictment with one count each of visa fraud, making false statements, acting as an agent of a foreign government and conspiracy. Ye is currently in China.

Zaosong Zheng, 30, a Chinese national, was arrested on Dec. 10, 2019, at Boston's Logan International Airport and charged by criminal complaint with attempting to smuggle 21 vials of biological research to China. On January 21, 2020, Zheng was indicted on one count of smuggling goods from the United States and one count of making false, fictitious, or fraudulent statements. He has been detained since December 30, 2019.

Based on recent published scientific papers, this new coronavirus has unique virologic features that suggest genetic engineering may have been involved in its creation. Dr. Yuhong Dong, who holds a doctorate in infectious disease from Beijing commented on a scientific paper published in *The Lancet* on January 30th, 2020. The paper in the concluding remarks states "...despite its occurrence, recombination is probably not the reason for emergence of this virus, although this inference might change if more closely related animal viruses are identified." It is anticipated that we will learn much more in the months ahead that will shine some light on the origin of this virus.

Dr. Yuhong brings up some other good points in the Lancet study by authors Roujian Lu et al., from China Key Laboratories of Biosafety, National Institute for Viral Disease Control and Prevention, Chinese Center for Disease Control and Prevention. They were that "...the outbreak was first reported in late December 2019, when most bat species in Wuhan are hibernating. Second, no bats were sold or found at the Huanan seafood market, whereas various non-aquatic animals (including mammals) were available for purchase. Third, the sequence identity between 2019-nCoV and its close bat-SL-CoVZC45 and bat-SLCoVZXC21 was less than 90%." This would indicate that these are not direct ancestors of the 2019-nCoV.

This strongly suggests that this is not a "wild virus" that jumped to humans from bats and raises very good questions regarding random mutation compared with engineered elements of the DNA. Once again Dr. Yuhong brings up some compelling questions. "How could this novel virus be so intelligent as to mutate precisely at selected sites while preserving its binding affinity to the human ACE2 receptor?

How did the virus change just four amino acids of the S-protein? Did the virus know how to use Clustered Regularly Interspaced Short Palindromic Repeats (CRISPR) to make sure this would happen?"

CRISPR is a cryptic acronym—or, to some ears, a drawer to keep lettuce fresh. Today, CRISPR Cas9, the most popular form of the powerful gene-editing technology, is widely used to accelerate experiments, grow pesticide-resistant crops, and design drugs to treat life-threatening genetic diseases like sickle cell anemia.

This puzzle becomes increasingly complex as we look over the research in this area. Many scientists around the world are now investigating the gene sequences found in the coronavirus, and they are increasingly concluding that elements of the virus have been engineered. Some scientists and researchers claim it couldn't happen by chance. They believe the coronavirus was not a random mutation in the wild but believe that it was engineered.

Many of those scientists are being threatened and censored. One paper has so far been forced to be withdrawn and revised, no doubt to remove the key conclusions that point to the genetic engineering origins of the coronavirus, but *the proof of its engineering cannot be denied forever.*

Furthermore, A recent interview with Bioweapons expert Dr. Francis Boyle published by *Great Game India* and conducted by *Geopolitics & Empire*, exploded across the globe early February 2020 as the truth is emerging on the origins of the Coronavirus Bioweapon.

Francis Boyle is a professor of international law at the University of Illinois College of Law. He drafted the U.S. domestic implementing legislation for the Biological Weapons Convention, known as the Biological Weapons Anti-Terrorism Act of 1989, that was approved unanimously by both Houses of the U.S. Congress and signed into law by President George H.W. Bush.

In an interview Dr Francis Boyle states:

> *It does seem to me that the Wuhan BSL-4 is the source of the coronavirus, yes. My guess is that they were researching SARS, and they weaponized it further by giving it gain-of-function*

properties, which means it could be more lethal, and indeed the latest report now is it's 15% fatality rate which is more than SARS, and 83% infection rate. So a typical gain-of-function is it travels in the air, so it could reach out maybe six feet or more from someone emitting a sneeze or a cough. Likewise, this is a specially designated WHO research lab, so the WHO is in on it, and they knew full well what was going on there.

Yes, it's also reported the Chinese stole coronavirus materials from the Canadian lab at Winnipeg; Winnipeg is Canada's foremost center for research developing and testing biological warfare weapons. It's along the lines of Ft. Detrick in the USA, and yeah, I have three degrees from Harvard, it would not surprise me if something was being stolen out of Harvard to turn over to China... the bottom line is, ... and I drafted the U.S. domestic implementing legislation for the biological weapons convention, that was approved unanimously by both houses of the U.S. Congress and signed into law by President Bush, Senior, that it appears the coronavirus that we're dealing with here is an offensive biological warfare weapon that leaked out of that Wuhan BSL-4 [lab]. *I'm not saying it was done deliberately, but there have been previous reports of problems with that lab and things leaking out of it, and I'm afraid that is what we are dealing with today. (Emphasis added)*[2]

More compelling information as well as curiously unanswered questions can be found in Appendix B.

Something else to consider is that the media states that this was picked up at a "wet market", selling strange animals like bats, snakes, or pangolins for human consumption. This statement as inferring that patrons of the market consumed contaminated animals who

---

2 In an enlightening interview with *Geopolitics and Empire*, Dr. Boyle reveals that the coronavirus now circulating in the wild, exploding as a pandemic, is indeed an "offensive biological warfare weapon."

contracted the virus and spread it. It is conceivable. but typically, highly unlikely that a virus is spread via the digestive system.

Bacteria *are* food-borne pathogens and are structured in such a way as to survive the digestive actions of hydrochloric acid in the stomach. For example, probiotics are bacteria that are able to withstand this environment and stay viable. Viruses on the other hand typically do not have such inherent protection from stomach acid. While food-borne viral infections are remotely possible, they are usually passed through body fluids and contracted by direct contact of these fluids. Contact with saliva, blood, feces, urine, vomit, semen, and mucus membranes are the standard routes of viral contraction. Coughing and sneezing are very efficient routes of contraction, as are the synthetic surfaces that harbor viral deposition. When you touch a contaminated surface such as a handle or counter top and then rub your eye or rub an itch on your nose, you can get infected, actions that one usually would not even register mentally which subsequently end up getting infected.

Let's continue to put this into perspective to give a better picture of what we are dealing with and why our local health officials are recommending certain measures. There are two measurements that help us get a feel for how quickly this will spread. The first is the R0 value (pronounced "R naught"). This is a mathematical calculation of how contagious a disease is, otherwise known as the reproduction number. The R0 is an equation which gives us some predictability of essentially how many people one infected person would transmit the disease to during the contagious stage of the disease. For example, if a disease has an R0 value of about 1 that means one person will pass it to another and so on. If it is greater than one, let's say 3 then the first generation would infect three people and the second generation would infect 9 and so forth.

Another helpful value is known as the Si or "serial interval." This represents the average time between the time of symptom onset of a primary case and that of a secondary case. This interval is widely used in infectious disease surveillance and control. If the Si is low then new cases will infect others more quickly and when the Si is higher it will take longer for the pathogen to incubate and subsequently infect others. In the case of CoVid-19 the Si is about 5-6 days compared to influenza which is 3 days. What this means is that influenza infections spread faster but since the R0 value is low the rate of infection is still fairly linear.

How we play with the numbers can tell a much different story. According to the CDC, the flu kills a surprising 3,300 to 49,000 people every year. This rather high number varies greatly in any given year, and according to many health experts is pretty exaggerated. Most years, US death certificates show fewer than 300 deaths attributed to the flu. A large issue in determining the actual number of flu-related deaths is differentiating the flu from other more serious illnesses with flu-like symptoms and those patients with underlying health conditions. The National Vital Statistics System reported fewer than 500 flu-related deaths in 2010—that's a lot less than the thousands of deaths estimated by the CDC. So how do these discrepancies occur? For one, without lab tests it's impossible to differentiate the real flu from more serious germs with flu-like symptoms. In 2001, 257 American death certificates listed the flu as cause of death. Only 18 of these 257 people were positively confirmed as having a true flu, while the remaining 239 were simply assumed to have died from the flu. The same inconsistency and manipulation of statistics seems to be used on a very broad scale with Covid-19. (O'Neil, 2020)

Let's clarify the difference between infectious and contagious. Basically, infectious diseases are caused by infectious agents (such as a virus or bacteria) while "contagious" refers to the type of infections that can be passed from person to person.

Contagious infections are spread either by touching or kissing the infected person, coming into contact with bodily fluids, or even touching an object they have touched. Other contagious illnesses may be airborne and are spread by infectious microbes released through talking, coughing, or sneezing. Infectious diseases are the second leading cause of death worldwide, and third in the United States. According to 2014 Tropical Medicine Reports, the

Dengue virus (DENV) is one of the most common viral diseases of the past 30 years, with approximately 390 million people infected globally each year. DENV is not a contagious illness and can't spread directly from person to person. According to information from the World Health Organization, people contract dengue fever if they are bitten by an infected female Aedes mosquito. In 2017, there were 80 reported cases of Dengue fever in the U.S. 43 of those were travel-related, and the 37 'local' contractions were in the US territories of American Samoa, Puerto Rico, and the Virgin Islands.

Just how contagious is SARS-CoV-2. I have heard some claims that it was fairly high. Let's look at the numbers of diseases many are familiar with or have at least heard about.

1. Hepatitis C. . . . . R0= 2
2. Seasonal Influenza. . R0= 2 (0.9 - 2.1)
3. HIV . . . . R0= 4 (2 - 4)
4. Measles. . . . . R0= 15 (12 - 18)
5. SARS-CoV-2 . . . . R0= 3 (1.4 - 3.9)

When the situation began and more cases were identified, the estimated number of deaths was much higher. Somewhere in the 5% – 7% range, however more recent figures have put it in the 2.3% range, according the figures gathered in late February and that number appears to be dropping significantly. Comparing this to SARS and MERS, it is more transmissible but less deadly.

On March 30th when I looked over the numbers the aggregated total was 781,390 worldwide and a death toll of 37,218. The US numbers were 163,479 total cases and 3,146 deaths. The numbers vary slightly depending on the reporting source.

As of April 3rd, 2020, the number of cases in the US is roughly 277,491 and the aggregate number of cases confirmed worldwide is 1,102,725. The number of deaths in the US is 7,144 and the world-wide total is 58,632. The number of cases in the US which have recovered is over 10,403. As of April 23rd 2020 the US numbers spiked to a total of 868,945 with a death toll of 49,887 and 80,174 recovered which means we are likely in the peak of the infection. Worldwide totals at this point were total cases 2,708,470 and a loss of 190,788. The number of recovered worldwide is 738,274.

Another look on August 12th 2020 shows the numbers have grown to over 5.1 million cases total and 3,310,105 active cases in the US and 163,651 deaths. Worldwide there are over 20.5 million cases with over 745,000 deaths. In the US the recovery reports count is over 1.8 million and worldwide over 12.6 million as recovered cases. Although projections vary from source to source with a variety of variable factors it looks like we are headed to have worldwide case counts well over 20 million and over 6 million in the US. Using current counts the death toll is about 0.5%. This should be a wakeup call and add perspective for preparing ourselves in the likely event of future outbreaks from other forms of Coronavirus or other more deadly pathogens.

To give CoVid-19 some reference the Spanish Flu (H1N1) circa 1918 killed nearly 100 million people worldwide. Tuberculosis kills around 1.5 million people worldwide every year, second only to malaria. Although past epidemics of Cholera have killed millions, currently it kills roughly 120,000 annually. Methicillin-resistant *Staphylococcus aureus* (MRSA) is considered a "Superbug" which is an antibiotic resistant bacteria with necrotizing (flesh eating) capabilities. Nearly 20,000 deaths due to MRSA and 55,000 due to influenza and pneumonia occur annually in the US.

The International Society of Travel Medicine on 28 February 2020 published in The Journal of Travel Medicine a study which helped get a better perspective of this phase of the disease. The name of the study was *"COVID-19 outbreak on the Diamond Princess cruise ship: estimating the epidemic potential and effectiveness of public health countermeasures"* which stated that the initial R0 estimation without intervention could have been as high as 14.8 which is about 4 times that of Wuhan due to the close quarters on the ship. However, due to the swift action the R0 value or rate of infection was reduced to 1.75, significantly lower.

In the CDC MMWR report of 27 March 2020 nearly one month later reported on the same incident showing the following conclusions. It is significant to note that this study grouped three cruise lines for the final outcome. These groups are separated in the body of the report. The Diamond Princess cruise line, which departed Yokohama, Japan carried 3711 passengers and crew. Of these 712 tested positive for SARS-Cov2 (19.2%) however, out of the group testing positive 331 (46.5%) were asymptomatic. Nearly half of the passengers testing positive exhibited no symptoms. Out of the symptomatic group 37 (9.7%) required intensive care and 9 passengers (1.3%) died as a result. Keep in mind that the median age was 52 and of those passengers that required higher level of intervention which tested positive several weeks later was 75 years.

Early in April Stanford University published an important study. In Santa Clara county 3,300 volunteers were tested for SARS-Cov2 virus. The conclusion of the study which correlated with the cruise line study shows that although the SARS-Cov2 is much more widespread than originally thought however, is less deadly than was projected. This study indicates 0.12% to 0.20% in contrast to the 3% that was reported weeks earlier. This study also shows that many people who tested positive were also asymptomatic. Although, not as many as initially projected had been exposed and thus, produced antibodies. We are seeing a much higher percentage of those that are non symptomatic with antibodies for SARS-Cov2.

USC ANTIBODY STUDY SHOWS CORONAVIRUS 'FAR MORE WIDESPREAD,' DEATH RATE 'MUCH LOWER.'

Preliminary research by USC and county finds 4.1% of county adults carry antibodies.

Recently an antibody study was released by USC and Los Angeles County Department of Health finding the novel coronavirus infection rate in Los Angeles County "far exceeds" the number of confirmed cases, meaning that the fatality rate is also "much lower" than previously thought.

The preliminary results of research conducted by USC and the Los Angeles County Department of Public Health found that about 4.1% of the county's adult population carries the SARS-Cov2 antibody, about 28 to 55 times higher than the 7,994 confirmed cases reported in early April.

Adjusted for the margin of error, the percentage of adults with the antibody ranges from 2.8% and 5.6%, which translates to between 221,000 and 442,000 adults. The county had recorded 617 deaths from the virus as of 20 April 2020. "These results indicate that many persons may have been unknowingly infected and at risk of transmitting the virus to others," said Dr. Barbara Ferrer, director of the public health department, in a press release.

A similar study released 17 April 2020 by Stanford University showed a similar phenomenon in Santa Clara County, finding that 2.8% to 4.2% of residents tested carrying antibody resistance to the virus, a percentage that far exceeded the number of recorded cases.

The same study posted in the USC News reports on testing results from 863 adults, the research team estimates that approximately 4.1% of the county's adult population has an antibody to the virus. Adjusting this estimate for the statistical margin of error implies about 2.8% to 5.6% of the county's adult population has an antibody to the virus—which translates to approximately 221,000 to 442,000 adults in the county who have been infected. That estimate is 28 to 55 times higher than the 7,994 confirmed cases of COVID-19 reported to the county at the time of the study in early April, 2020. The number of COVID-related deaths in the county has now surpassed 600.

Miami-Dade has tens of thousands of missed coronavirus infections, UM survey finds. Roughly 6% of Miami-Dade's population—about 165,000 residents—have antibodies indicating a past infection by the novel coronavirus, dwarfing the state health department's tally of about 10,600 cases. (According to preliminary study results announced by University of Miami on 24 April 2020)

The study, spurred by Miami-Dade County officials, will be an ongoing weekly survey based on antibody testing—randomly selecting county residents to volunteer pinpricks of their blood to be screened for signs of a past COVID-19 infection, whether they had tested positive for the virus in the past or not. The goal is to measure the extent of infection in the community.

Friday's results (April 24, 2020); based on two weeks of county-wide antibody testing and about 1,400 participants, found that about half of the people who tested positive for antibodies reported no symptoms in the 14-17 days before being tested. If the trend holds, the findings could have major implications for understanding not only the number of people infected, but also how many have symptoms and, in turn, how the virus spreads.

Although, these studies give us better projections which will allow us to begin opening things up, it also indicates that we are not out of the woods yet. There are some variables yet to be determined. How long is the immunity that our body has once exposed? When will we reach the herd immunity critical mass and probably the most disturbing is how will this virus mutate and what will that look like? Our best defense even if a vaccine was ready for testing would be strengthening your own inherent immune function. Admittedly vaccines carry with them very serious hazards as is reflected by the Vaccine Injury Act of 1986. The quicker you are to act at giving your body the tools it needs in the form of proper nutrition, lowered stress, adequate sleep, and a balanced nerve system; the sooner you will be prepared to win a war you may not see coming

CHAPTER THREE
PROTECT YOURSELF: TAKE CARE OF YOUR FAMILY

An ounce of prevention is worth a pound of cure.

— Benjamin Franklin

Miriam had just returned from a small town in Brazil where she spent the first eight years of her life. Her description of life there was certainly not what you would see in a travel magazine. There was a large disparity between those that had the basic comforts we enjoy and the average citizens struggling to ensure the consumption of the next meal and a safe place to sleep. The people were very nice, but as you walked around town, it was important to stay on guard. The pick pockets were swift, and the thugs would steal the shoes off your feet. People lived as if they would have to head for the hills on a moment's notice if the political climate changed. Who you once thought was in power could possibly become an outlaw.

This was going through my head as I saw things change in my own town here in Orange County, California. People started to get very worried as word got around that toilet paper was becoming scarce. People stocked up as if it were some rare commodity. Within days the shelves on most of the markets were bare as panic swept the area.

What would you be willing to do to feed or protect your family? If, in fact, a situation or crises broke out, would you be truly prepared to do what it took to make sure you and those you care about made it through?

I hope to shine some light on how you can prepare yourself. This is not intended to be a comprehensive list but rather a broad brush stroke inventory of factors that I would encourage you to consider in preparation for various types of crisis situations. Also keep in mind, this is a gradual scale of preparedness. Take one step, even if it's small, and build from there.

When things go wrong what is your mindset? Are you the hunter or the hunted? The predator or the prey?

When a situation arises or a crisis hits, this is the time, more than ever, that a community should stay together and connected. The elderly and those with chronic medical conditions can be at increased risk when it comes to infection by the CoVid-2019 coronavirus. Check in on your loved ones and vulnerable community members to ensure they have what is needed to get through and that they are safe. Keep each other informed and consider sharing this information with your community. A well informed and prepared community is better equipped to weather the storm.

The late Colonel Cooper designed a color code chart that associated levels of awareness to specific colors. Cooper was a USMC firearms instructor. He broke down situational awareness into four levels of escalating degrees of preparation for police use of deadly force.

This system is a mental process, not a physical one, and should be utilized whether or not you are armed—though, in my opinion, being armed is preferred. Being alert may help you to avoid a deadly threat in the first place, which is always the preferred outcome. Being alert can buy you time and time can buy you options.

Condition White represents a state of complete unawareness and unpreparedness. In this state you are oblivious to things going on around you and are exceedingly vulnerable to attack.

Condition Yellow represents a state of relaxed alert. There is no specific, obvious threat present, but you are aware that danger is always a possibility. You are aware of people around you as well as the environment in general.

Condition Orange is a heightened state of awareness in which you observe or are aware of a specific threat. In this condition, you are beginning to formulate possible responses to deal with the danger. An example of this is when you realize that a threat is indeed following you or advancing toward you.

Condition Red is the stage associated with action, when things have escalated to the point where you are either engaging a threat or are in retreat. It is physically and mentally exhausting to be in Condition Red, as it demands that you be 100-percent dedicated to the danger at hand.

The preferred state of daily operation would be level yellow. Keeping aware of one's surroundings can help you avoid many troubles.

Planning is the first step in being prepared. This sounds logical, but it is so often left for the last minute. I have heard many people say, "Oh that will never happen," or "If this or that occurs, then I will get some supplies."

Recently during the panic over the coronavirus, many experienced the difficulty shopping for some of the basic staple items such as toilet paper, water, hand sanitizer as well as many food items, producing long lines at the store. Store shelves emptied in a panic for those seeking supplies at the last minute. The turbulent experience produced high levels of stress.

As the fear began to wane with Covid-19 and communities began to move toward a more normal operation of activities civil unrest gained momentum over the George Floyd incident. On May 25th, 2020 in Minneapolis, Minnesota Floyd's altercation with police, which was mishandled and unfortunately resulted in his death, sparked a wildfire of protests across the country. In some areas the backlash resulted in looting and rioting, creating unstable and unsafe areas across the US.

Now is the time to get prepared for an unpredictable event such as those we have recently experienced. Undoubtedly we will experience others in the future. It is not a matter of "IF" but a matter of "WHEN" and "WHERE." These situations can arise at any moment and can take on many different forms. Although it would be difficult to attempt to cover all scenarios I have taken a broad look at sharing some basics to point you in the right direction.

Here's a list of items you may need during an emergency situation. The first 25 items usually go first during a crisis situation, so you may want to keep them on hand. These also may vary slightly as climate change or area may influence these factors.

1. Generators (Good ones can be expensive. It can be a target for thieves due to the noise)

2. Water

3. Water Filters/Purifiers

4. Portable Toilet

5. Seasoned Firewood. Wood takes about 6-12 months to be ready for home use.

6. Lamp Oil, Wicks, Lamps (Buy clear oil. If scarce, stockpile)

7. Coleman Fuel

8. Charcoal and Lighter fluid

9. Family Protection (guns, ammunition, pepper spray, knives)

10. Cooking utensils (hand can opener, whisk, etc)

11. Honey/sugar/syrups

12. Rice/beans/ wheat

13. Vegetable oil (for cooking)

14. Water containers (get more than one and in different sizes)

15. Propane Heaters and all accessories that go with it (extra propane, heads, etc)

16. Fishing accessories (line, hooks, bobbies, etc)

17. Lighting sources - short term and long term (flashlights, hurricane lamps, etc)

18. Batteries

19. Basin to do laundry in/wash boards, etc

20. Cook stoves

21. Vitamins

22. Thermal underwear (top and bottoms)

23. Tools (bow saw, axes, hatchets, wedges (honing oil)

24. Aluminum Foil

25. Propane Cylinder Handle-Holder (Small canister use is dangerous without this item)

We can categorize supplies into several categories which may help you prepare. Keep in mind that these supplies may vary depending on the situation and your plan. I suggest breaking up your supplies into various quantities for the following situations.

1. If you had to leave your home on foot or were caught away from home, have enough supplies on hand that you could carry and live off of for several days or perhaps a week or two. Keep in mind if you had to carry these they need to be packed light enough that you could move fast and still carry your supplies. Staying in

shape helps with this so it is important to have a good exercise program in place now.

2. If it's necessary to stay home for several weeks or even a month, have enough essentials on hand.

3. If you have time to pack a vehicle and leave your home, consider what you can load into your car and where you will go?

CONSIDER THE SUPPLIES YOU WILL NEED.

1. For survival
   a. Food and food storage (including animals if you have them)

   b. Water, water purification and storage

   c. First Aid and Skills (including medications)

   d. Security and protection

   e. Communications

   f. Shelter

   g. Sanitation which includes items for both genders.

2. For sanity
   a. Keep in mind this will be a stressful situation. You may want some comfort foods, coffee, tea, chocolate etc.

   b. a deck of cards or some easy to pack games

   c. a couple books etc.

3. For bartering
   a. Have some cash on hand in smaller denominations, as ATM's, credit cards etc. may not be an option.

b. If you have the space and time to have plenty of certain items on hand this could come in very handy. Comfort foods, regular foods, water and hygiene items.

The CoVid-19 outbreak has caused significant concern on many levels. Along with the outbreak itself the economic implications are unsettling to many. The more prepared you can be the less stressful the situation. Here is a more simplified but complete list for the current situation as it stands at the time of this writing. The WHO declared Covid-19 a pandemic in January which was later upgraded to "global pandemic" more on this in appendix C.

FOOD

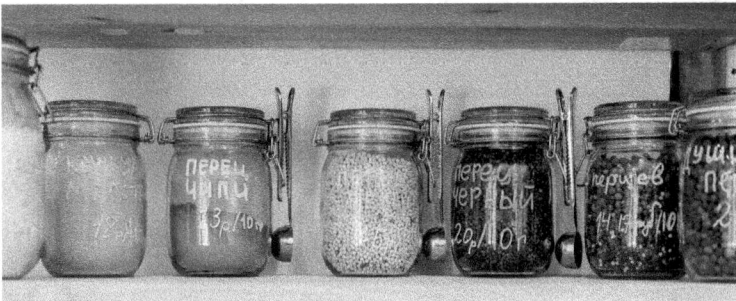

Fill the freezer

Frozen vegetables such as spinach, broccoli, cauliflower, carrots

1. Frozen berries
2. Animal protein such as fish, chicken, grass-fed beef
3. Stock the pantry
4. Protein powders
5. Electrolyte replacement
6. Greens powder
7. Canned or dry beans and lentils
8. Canned oysters, sardines

9. Pasta sauce
10. Dry noodles
11. Vegetable broth
12. Nuts and seeds
13. Grains such as rice, quinoa, oats
14. Coconut milk
15. Olive oil
16. Coffee & herbal teas
17. Applesauce
18. Crackers
19. Bottled water - You may consider minimizing plastics and use glass or stainless steel when possible or at least get BPA safe material. Keeping well hydrated will help keep you healthy.

Don't forget about the pets! Have an additional bag of food and extra water on hand to ensure the animals stay well-fed.

MEDICINE CABINET

Supportive supplements (This is not a comprehensive list, always check with your healthcare provider)

1. Multivitamin
2. Vitamin D
3. Vitamin C (Natural or Mineral Chelated)
4. Zinc
5. Omega-3 (fish oil)
6. Refill any recommended supplements you are currently taking
7. Thymus support
8. Echinacea

Over-the-counter and prescription medications (This is not a comprehensive list, always check with your healthcare provider)

1. Antihistamine
2. Decongestant
3. Ibuprofen
4. Refill any prescribed medications you are currently taking

First aid

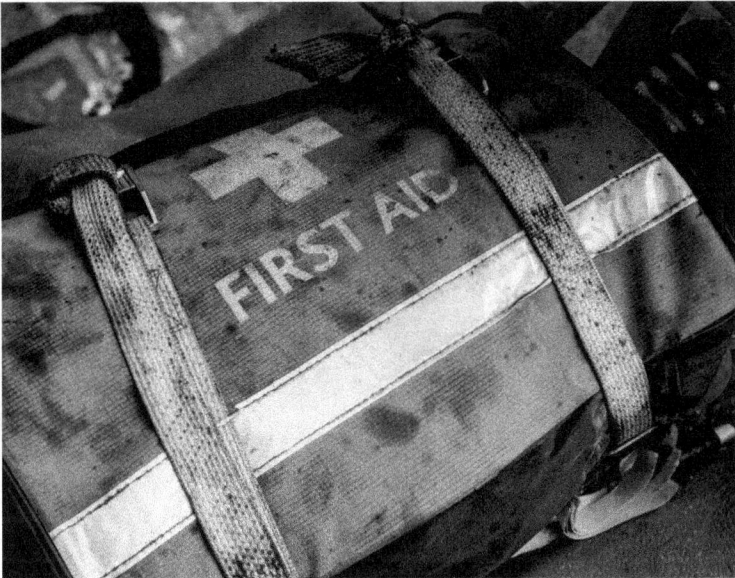

1. Adhesive bandages
2. Hand sanitizer
3. Hydrogen peroxide
4. Scissors
5. Adhesive tape
6. Bandages
7. Gauze
8. Quikclot gauze
9. CAT Tourniquet

HOUSEHOLD ITEMS

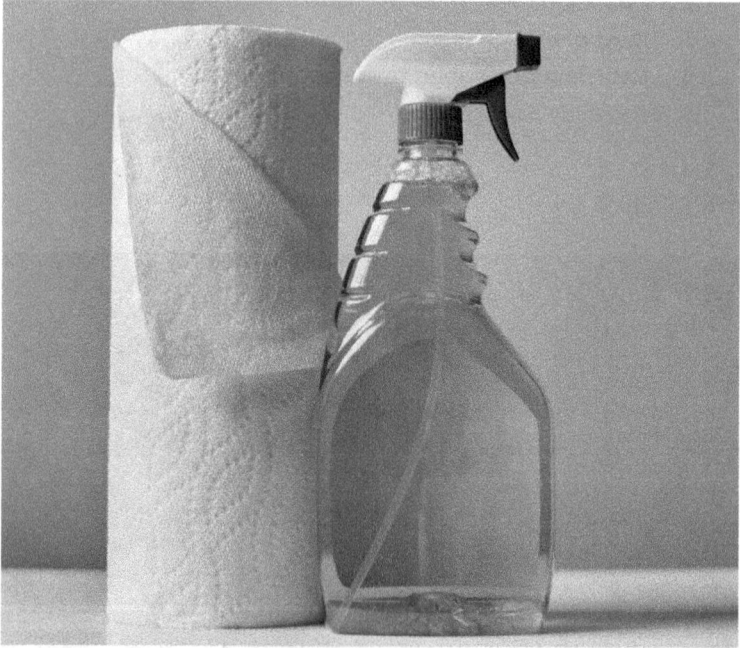

Cleaning products

1. Hand soap
2. Laundry and dish detergent
3. Disinfectant wipes

Personal care

1. Body wash, shampoo
2. Toothpaste and toothbrushes
3. Sanitary products
4. Toilet paper and facial tissue

Additional items

1. Flashlight + extra batteries
2. Extra cash

3. Can opener
4. Battery-operated radio + batteries
5. Books and puzzles

If you are confined to your home or other location for extended periods of time, have your favorite books, movies, puzzles or games. Make a list of those projects you always wanted "To Do" that you never had time?

If you think you might be sick with the CoVid-19, stay home and call your health care provider for advice. For those who are elderly or have a significant chronic medical condition, it's important to avoid crowds. Eat healthy, get enough sleep, and exercise to reduce stress and maintain good health.

CHAPTER FOUR

STAY CALM—THE SOLUTION IS CLOSER THAN YOU THINK

Beyond drama and chaos, beyond anxiety and fear, lies a zone of endless peace and love. Let's all take a very deep breath, slow down for just a moment and remember this. That alone will open the door.

—Marianne Williamson

In the first several weeks as the pandemic swept across the United States, uncertainly along with misconceptions fed into a storm of anxiety which quickly went ablaze. Tom and Delilah embarked on their typical end of the week shopping and were surprised when the shelves that once contained paper products such as toilet paper, paper towels, and hand wipes were stripped bare. Luckily for them, they had a small supply of these things. It was a mystery as to why those particular items were in such a demand.

As the next several weeks would prove it didn't getting any better. Lines at the markets were growing and the shelves were stripped bare. One interesting observation was that many of the perishable food items were in good supply. Although for most of the people, the N95 masks would prove to be unnecessary, but they were soon sold out. Many wore them for peace of mind.

Tom remarked as he watched a man wearing gloves. "He's touching random objects and still touching his face with the gloves, and then he takes the gloves off and puts them into his pocket, as if the gloves had some special power to give viral protection."

Delilah stood patiently on one of the blue tape lines to enter the store which would only allow a certain number of shoppers in at one time. She and Tom found comfort in knowing they had taken some Vitamin C, Echinacea, and Zinc as part of the daily routine, along with a visit to the Chiropractor that week. They knew that keeping the immune system strong was a person's best defense against a pathogen including SARS-CoV-2.

Your most powerful weapon against this and other biological threats is your own immune system. This virus, as is the case with others, can spread rapidly and survive for extended periods of time on a surface without a host. You can be asymptomatic during incubation period but the virus can be transmitted during this time. Specialized testing is required to detect it.

Let's take a closer look at the SARS-CoV-2 so we have a clear picture of what we are addressing. The SARS-CoV-2 is an airborne virus. This means that depending on the size of the pathogen, it either floats around in the air just as dust would or it is carried on small particulate matter that moves through the air. In the case of the SARS-CoV-2, due to its size, it typically will not float around, but rather is carried by droplets such as saliva or a discharge from the nose as in sneezing. Without a host, it is not likely to live more than a few hours in the air. The virus can also live on a surface for varying amounts of time.

Your best defense is minimizing exposure and improving your immune function. Stress will not help the situation so reducing your stress is important. This can take the form of taking walks outside, listening to music, dancing, exercise, yoga, meditation, supplements for stress and adrenal support etc. Since laughter can be a powerful tool in decreasing stress, incorporate humor when possible.

As with any crisis, it is important to get correct information and keep things in perspective. The best way to encourage children to follow good habits is to lead by example. Take the time to teach children how to act during these turbulent times and encourage them to share this information with others.

Here are some practical guidelines for minimizing exposure.

SOCIAL DISTANCING

The more you can minimize contact with others, the less chance you will have in contracting the disease. The virus is usually spread from person-to-person when infected people are in close contact with one another (within about 6 feet) usually confined areas such as elevators, busy malls, airports, bus stations etc. Infection occurs through respiratory droplets produced when an infected person coughs or sneezes. It does not float around in the air. It is highly unlikely a person would become infected by being outside. In fact getting outside and engaging in some exercise will actually reduce your risk.

These droplets can land in the mouths or noses of people who are nearby or possibly be inhaled into the lungs. The droplets can also enter via the eyes. If you do not have to travel, then stay home. When shopping for necessities, shop during nonpeak hours. Make an effort to know who you are coming in contact with and keep that circle of people to a minimum. Older people should stay away from younger people as well as minimize contact with others as much as possible. Those over 60 or those with heart disease, diabetes, and lung disease are considered high risk according to the CDC.

An unfortunate development from all of this is the decrease of contact. Shaking hands and the giving of hugs has been greatly discouraged. Social distancing seems to be almost an oxymoron of the time. Some alternatives to shaking hands are tapping elbows, tapping feet, or even tapping hips. I find that the language we use also has an effect on us. Perhaps rather than using "social distancing" we consider "physically distancing" while we remain socially interactive.

WHY SEVERE SOCIAL DISTANCING MIGHT ACTUALLY RESULT IN MORE CORONAVIRUS DEATHS

What the media and policymakers are not telling us is that the longer we delay the development of herd immunity, the more elderly or high-risk people will become infected and die.

Many doctors and immunologists argue about the best strategy for addressing this tragic public health crisis. Many experts agree with the Imperial College Covid19 Response Team, their information was summarized well in an article by Hillsdale College. Data from these studies, received as of April 2020, can be used to better serve the health and welfare of the community. Despite the inherent risks of a vaccine stated by the manufacturer, which I would encourage you to read, researchers state that the development of one with even some efficacy would be 12 - 18 months away. Doing nothing would be overwhelming to the health care system and potential more deaths due to delayed intervention. However, the projections also show that if we excessively restrict public movement and restrain interaction too stringently, it will flatten the curve to a degree that will prolong herd immunity[1] and would have a damaging effect economically. In addition, heightened amounts of restricted activity and the reopening of public areas before herd immunity is reached will inevitably lead to an increase of COVID-19 cases.

The best method, offering a quick path to herd immunity without straining the healthcare system nor economy, is to take a milder approach to physical distancing. This approach would include limiting crowds to no more than 30 to 50 at a time, temporary closure of schools, and voluntary isolation of those who would be at higher risk. This procedure in the community would aid the increase of herd immunity faster with limited economic burden. "Why?" you may ask would it cause more deaths to have stricter isolation standards? Because it is typically the young and healthy that contribute to the herd immunity effect in most cases, by having stricter isolation, we greatly prolong the time for herd immunity to take effect.

[3]Herd immunity is achieved when a certain percentage of the community has been exposed to the pathogen, this is generally seen as 60% - 70% by most experts in this field.

---

3 Herd immunity is achieved when a certain percentage of the community has been exposed to the pathogen, this is generally seen as 60% - 70% by most experts in this field.

CLEAN HANDS

Wash your hands often with soap and water for at least 20 seconds, especially after you have been in a public place, or after blowing your nose, coughing, or sneezing, as well as before meals and after using the toilet. You may also consider washing after being exposed to a high traffic area such as a store, airport, or other busy place. Be sure to get all the areas, rub your hands under running water for a full 20–30 seconds. If you don't have soap, but you have water, wash your hands anyway in as hot a water as you can take. Washing your hands with water alone has been shown to be almost as effective as washing your hands with soap. On the other hand, I recommend using soap with essential oils, which are antiviral. Dry your hands using a clean cloth or a disposable towel.

Keep in mind the skin is the largest organ in the body. The skin helps regulate body temperature and water retention. Not only does it trap or release heat to help keep you warm or cool depending on the temperature outside, the nerve endings in the skin also help you feel if a surface is too hot or cold or other sensations like pressure and pain.

But the skin's most apparent job is to act as a barrier. As your first line of defense, skin prevents germs and the sun's ultraviolet rays from entering the body. Microorganisms living on the skin protect the body from invasion of more harmful bacteria or viruses. The skin microbiota may also communicate with T cells, which are active players in the body's immune response, preparing them to respond to harmful organisms the skin may encounter in the future.

Keeping your skin healthy plays a large role in keeping your body healthy. Eating a healthy diet and taking care of the skin will have an effect on your immune system's first line of defense. The skin's microbiome flourishes under a more acidic environment. A low pH level is a measure of acidity (0 being most acidic and a high value of 14 being most basic). On average, the pH of the skin's surface is below 5. Topical products such as soaps, sanitizers, and moisturizes can disrupt and raise that ideal pH level of the skin.

Alcohol-based hand sanitizers may not be the panacea for hand hygiene. Mounting research indicates they may not be effective substitutes for soap and water. In some cases they may actually increase the risk for outbreaks of highly contagious viruses in health care settings. Many hand sanitizers contain toxic ingredients such as Tricolsan which the FDA has acknowledged as causing hormonal disruption.

Staff in facilities that experienced norovirus outbreaks were six times more likely to use hand sanitizers equally or more than soap and water for routine hand hygiene, according to the study (*American Journal of Infection Control* 2011;39:296–301). Of 45 facilities that reported preferential use of alcohol-based hand sanitizers, 53% experienced a confirmed outbreak of norovirus, compared with 18% of 17 facilities that used hand sanitizers less often than soap and water.

A more healthy approach is the use of a natural soap and essential oils. An article in the *American Journal of Essential Oils and Natural Products* suggests that some essential oils may help fight viruses. The study strongly suggested the following essential oils have shown some antiviral activity: bergamot oil, eucalyptus oil, red thyme, and cinnamon leaf. As well, some scientists suggest Tea Tree oil may also have antiviral properties if a person incorporates it into air filtering systems. Clove has high antiviral properties. Lemon balm may contain ingredients that could help prevent one type of bird flu virus from reproducing, according to one laboratory study.

- If soap and water are not readily available, use a hand sanitizer that contains at least 60% alcohol. Cover all surfaces of your hands and rub them together until they feel dry. On the other hand, I personally recommend using a more natural soap with essential oils which are antiviral. More on this in the next section. Note: alcohol is not quite as effective as hand washing.

- Avoid touching your eyes, nose, and mouth with unwashed hands. Most people touch their faces 23 times an hour! Your face contains mucous membranes, which are susceptible to entry by viruses, including the novel coronavirus. Because mucous membranes are especially susceptible to viruses, it's important that you keep your hands away from these mucous membranes— which include your eyes, your nose, and your mouth. An alternative would be to use a tissue, or perhaps a pen to scratch that itch.

- As we go through our daily lives we come into contact with many surfaces. These surfaces can be the perfect resting place for a whole host of viruses, bacteria and even chemicals.

SURFACES

Be aware of the following: doorknobs and door handles, handrails, elevator buttons, ATMs, grocery store checkout keypads, electronic signature capture pens, public electronic tablets and touch screens, water fountains and water cooler buttons, car surfaces in cars that are exposed to the public, especially cars serving in ride-sharing services like Uber and Lyft, almost anything at an airport, mall or high traffic area including arm rests and touch screens.

You can also use a tissue, paper towel and even a shirt sleeve if you must. As you disinfect your home or office pay particular attention to the door knobs and door handles, tables, drawers, handles, light switches, facets, countertops, toilets, keys, especially house keys and car keys, refrigerator handles, phones both mobile and landlines, popular containers within the refrigerator, charging cords for electronic devices that get touched often, remote controls, thermostats, electronic tablets and any other item prone to being touched or in the line of spray if someone were to sneeze in that area.

In some situations, you may consider wearing gloves. Nonsterile disposable patient examination gloves, which are used for routine patient care in healthcare settings, are appropriate for the care of patients with suspected or confirmed COVID-19. Gloves can give a person a false sense of security. If worn properly they are very effective. They should not be put on, taken off, and then put back on. This opens up the possibility of infection. Keep in mind that when you don gloves and touch an object which is potentially contaminated; throw the gloves away when you are done. I see many people wearing gloves and holding their cell phone, adjusting their glasses and touching there face. This type of use does NOT offer you any protection. Use common sense if you are going to use gloves. Imagine you put gloves on and then dip your hand in wet paint or your dog just left a mess and you cleaned it using your gloved hands. How then would you use those gloved hands? You would not touch any surface that you were concerned could be contaminated. Chances are that you would not take off the gloves and put them in your pocket.

Cover your mouth and nose with a tissue when you cough or sneeze or use the inside of your elbow. I actually feel that using the inside of your elbow is ridiculous, if you were actually infected this would promote the spread as it is unlikely one would disinfect the inside of their elbow. I suggest using your hands and then washing them in with soap and water. Science has shown sneezes travel up to 93 miles per hour and smaller particles cover distances up to 200 feet.

Throw used tissues in the trash. Immediately wash your hands with soap and water for at least 20 seconds. If soap and water are not readily available, clean your hands with a hand sanitizer that contains at least 60% alcohol or even better an alcohol, essential oil blend.

FACEMASKS

If you are sick, you should wear a facemask when around other people (e.g. sharing a room or vehicle) and before you enter a healthcare provider's office. If you are not able to wear a facemask because it causes trouble breathing, then you should do your best to cover your coughs and sneezes. People who are caring for you should wear a facemask when they enter your room. There is also no need to wear a mask while driving or in your own home unless, of course, you are caring or transporting someone that is infected.

If you are going to use a mask, there is a distinct difference between a mask and a respirator. These also have different ratings. Masks help protect the sterile field and reduce large particles. They are designed to protect the patient from the exhaled microorganisms from the healthcare provider.

Respirators in contrast meet the CDC Guidelines for *Mycobacterium tuberculosis* exposure control. They are certified by NIOSH as N95's and designed to provide a secure face-to-respirator seal. This seal helps reduce the wearer's exposure to airborne particles.

The mask of choice as long as you do not have a breathing problem is the N95 respirator. This is a respiratory protective device designed to achieve a very close facial fit and very efficient filtration of airborne particles.

The 'N95' designation means that when subjected to careful testing, the respirator blocks at least 95 percent of very small (0.3 micron) test particles and the N means that it is not resistant to oil. If properly fitted, the filtration capabilities of N95 respirators exceed those of face masks. However, even a properly fitted N95 respirator does not completely eliminate the risk of illness or death.

If you are NOT sick: You do not need to wear a facemask unless you are caring for someone who is sick and they are not able to wear a facemask. Facemasks may be in short supply and should be saved for caregivers. The Centers for Disease Control and Prevention (CDC) does not recommend that the general public wear N95 respirators to protect themselves from respiratory diseases, including coronavirus (COVID-19). Realize that contrary to many recommendations, most of the home-made masks are of minimal benefit, unless the individual is actually sick. Additionally, the infection typically will enter via mucus membranes such as the nose and mouth. However, it can also easily enter through the eye and tear duct if you happened to come into contact with particulate matter recently sprayed in the air from a cough or sneeze. If you are in a space that is highly suspicious of contamination, protective eye wear would also be necessary.

Clean AND disinfect frequently touched surfaces daily. This includes tables, doorknobs, light switches, countertops, handles, desks, phones, keyboards, toilets, faucets, and sinks. If surfaces are dirty, clean them: Use detergent or soap and water prior to disinfection.

Here's a couple of options for making your own solutions. You can add essential oils to these solutions as well and use less of the harsher ingredients.

Dilute Your Household Bleach

To make a bleach solution, mix:

- 5 tablespoons (1/3rd cup) bleach per gallon of water

OR

- 4 teaspoons bleach per quart of water

Follow manufacturer's instructions for application and proper ventilation. Check to ensure the product is not past its expiration date. Never mix household bleach with ammonia or any other cleanser. Unexpired household bleach will be effective against coronaviruses when properly diluted.

Alcohol Solutions

Insure the solution has at least 70% alcohol. There are many DIY recipes available for making your own disinfectant spray. Here is a simple and effective one:

Pour one cup of rubbing alcohol into a clean, empty spray bottle. Add 15 drops of Tea Tree EO, 7 drops of Lemon EO and 7 drops of Lavender EO. Mix well.

You may also use combinations of the following oils. I have included some of the most common and useful oils with a little background on each.

ESSENTIAL OILS

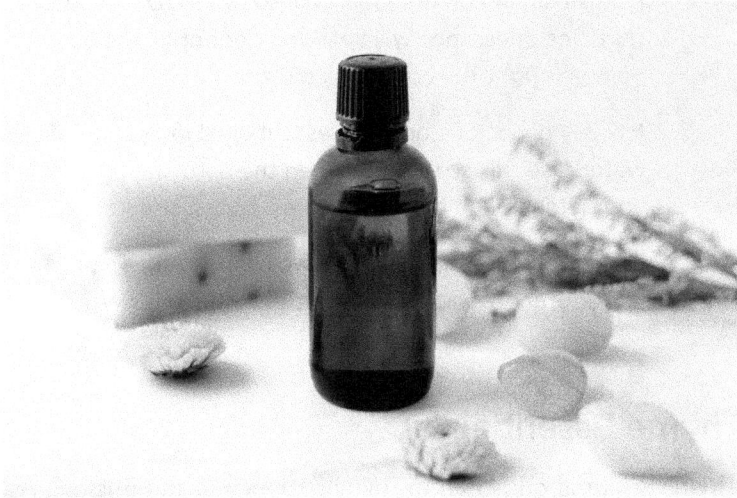

Cinnamon Essential Oil

Cinnamon essential oil has beautiful sweet and spicy aroma that can be used for deodorizing and purifying air at home.

Cinnamon essential oil is not only known for its pleasing scent but for its powerful antibacterial mechanisms as well. The rise of drug-resistant bacteria has forced the medicine to start exploring and embracing the antibacterial activity of cinnamon essential oil.

In 2018 a study published in the Microbial Pathogenesis (panelYueWangaYiZhangbYan-qinShiaXian-huaPanaYan-hua-LubPingCaoc, 2018), found cinnamon essential oil and its two constituents called cinnamaldehyde and cinnamic acid successfully inhibit bacteria by damaging their cell membrane.

Once the membrane is destroyed, all cell processes and motility of given microbe are altered. Using cinnamon essential oil in your daily cleaning routine will help you kill those stubborn, disease-causing germs.

TIPS FOR USE:

1. Diffuse cinnamon essential oil into the air. Dispersed particles of essence will help you deodorize the air and help you fight the common cold and flu.

2. Mix 3-4 drops of cinnamon essential oil in 1 gallon of water. Use this solution to clean the hard surfaces of your kitchen and bathroom (tiles, floors, sinks etc.)

3. Cinnamon essential oil mixes well with ylang-ylang, sweet orange, and peppermint essential oils.

Thyme Essential Oil

Thyme essential oil is rich in thymol, carvacrol, and linalool. All these constituents will help you stay protected from bacteria and other environmental threats, even those found in food. Salmonella, for instance, is a bacteria genus that often contaminates eggs, poultry, and other raw meats. According to the *International Journal of Food Microbiology*, thyme essential oil is potent enough to inhibit the salmonella.

In addition, a recent study published in the *Journal of Food and Drug Analysis* determined that thyme essential oil can be used as a natural food preservative due to its high anti-fungal and antibacterial activities. If thyme essential oil is safe enough for food, then it surely is safe enough to be used as a non-toxic cleaner for your home.

TIPS FOR USE:

1. Thyme essential oil blends well with lavender, oregano, grapefruit, and rosemary essential oils.

2. Clean your kitchen utensils, dishes, and chopping boards with homemade thyme essential oil dish soap after they have been in contact with poultry or any other raw meat.

Thyme Essential Oil Dish Soap

INGREDIENTS:

- ¼ cup castile soap
- ¼ cup soap flakes
- 2 teaspoons super washing soda
- 1 teaspoon vegetable glycerin
- 2 cups of water
- 30 drops of thyme essential oil

INSTRUCTIONS:

- Dissolve soap flakes in boiling water.

- Add other ingredients to the mix.

- Stir well and make sure everything is dissolved and well combined.

- Pour the liquid into a pump bottle.

- Leave 24 hours to set.

If the soap is too thick, add a little bit more water to it, and if it is too runny, heat it up once again and add more washing soda to it.

Tea Tree Essential Oil

Tea tree essential oil is a staple cleaning product in many households. Due to its purifying properties, Tea Tree oil can be found as an ingredient in many skincare products and shampoos. It cleanses the skin and purifies the air.

Research published in the *Physical Chemistry Chemical Physics* showed that tea tree oil in combination with eucalyptus essential oil was successful at fighting staph infection and E. coli. Both essential oils caused the microbes to leak their vital fluids.

A number of medical studies point to the powerful antibacterial and antiviral qualities of tea tree oil. This essential oil can be used as a household cleaner and as a treatment for various infections, from athlete's foot to cold sores and warts.

TIPS FOR USE:

1. Add 1-2 drops of tea tree oil to a teaspoon of coconut oil or raw honey. Use this balm to disinfect and treat the affected areas on your skin.

2. Diffuse few drops of tea tree oil to purify and sanitize the air in your home.

3. Tea tree oil blends well with lemon, lavender, and ylang-ylang essential oils.

4. Clean any hard surfaces in your home with this all-purpose tea tree oil cleaner.

All-Purpose Tea Tree Oil Cleaner

INGREDIENTS:

- 3 cups of water
- ½ cup of apple cider vinegar
- 10 drops of tea tree essential oil

INSTRUCTIONS:

- Add all ingredients to a spray bottle and shake well.

- Use this cleaner on floors, sinks, and countertops.

Toilet Bowel Scrub

Try disinfecting your toilet with a homemade toilet bowel scrub.

INGREDIENTS:

- 1 cup vinegar
- ½ cup baking soda
- ½ teaspoon tea tree essential oil

INSTRUCTIONS:

- Mix vinegar and essential oil in a glass spray bottle.

- Spray the inside and the outside of your toilet with the solution. Let it sit for a couple of minutes.

- Evenly distribute baking soda on the surface and start scrubbing it with a toilet brush.

- Use a dry or damp cloth to wipe down the toilet seat.

Oregano Essential Oil

Oregano essential oil is rich with bactericidal phenols that can help you improve your cleaning routine. You can also substitute your store-bought bathroom chemical cleaners with oregano essential oil. The potent essence of oregano is strong enough to inhibit E. coli and bacterium called Pseudomonas aeruginosa. This germ is mostly found in hot tubs, pools and other standing water as well as on the objects that are regularly exposed to moisture.

Oregano essential oil can disinfect and refresh the nooks and crannies of your bathroom and your kitchen. Antiseptic nature of oregano will help you keep harmful E. coli out of the kitchen.

TIPS FOR USE:

1. Diffuse oregano essential oil into the air. Dispersed oregano essence will help you refresh your home and fight the symptoms of seasonal respiratory illnesses.

2. Oregano mixes well with other antiseptic essential oils especially tea tree, rosemary, and lavender essential oils.

3. Disinfect your bathroom and kitchen with this all-purpose oregano oil cleaner.

All-Purpose Oregano Essential Oil Cleaner

INGREDIENTS:

- 2 cups of water
- 2 teaspoons of castile soap
- 20-30 drops of oregano essential oil

INSTRUCTIONS:

- Mix all ingredients in a glass spray bottle.

- Feel free to substitute oregano essential oil with a mix of different essential oils.

- Use this solution to clean your shower, kitchen countertop, and trash cans.

- Keep the cleaner in cool, dark place.

Peppermint Essential Oil

Peppermint essential oil is a terrific natural cleaning agent. Its impressive antiseptic properties can be attributed to the constituent called menthol. Menthol is an active ingredient covering up to 60% of the oil's chemical composition.

Such potent antibacterial formula can be used for disinfecting surfaces and repelling insects, such as spiders, ants, mosquitoes, and cockroaches. Fresh minty aroma of peppermint will help you purify your home and keep it free of creepy crawlies.

The use of peppermint oil cleaner for sanitizing your bathroom is highly recommended. According to the 2017 study published in the *Journal of Applied Microbiology*, peppermint oil showed the best antibacterial activity against *C. difficile* out of all tested processed products. *C. difficile* is a bacterium that thrives in toilets, bathing tubs, and other objects that may be in contact with feces. Healthcare providers are often transmitters of this germ.

TIPS FOR USE:

1. Diffuse peppermint essential oil into the air. Microscopic peppermint particles will purify the air and repel mosquitoes.

2. In a spray bottle, mix 10 drops of peppermint essential oil with a cup of water. Use this spray to wipe down hard surfaces in your home.

3. Peppermint essential oil mixes well with lemongrass, tea tree, lavender, and eucalyptus essential oils.

4. Use this all-purpose peppermint spray for deep cleaning.

All-Purpose Peppermint Spray

INGREDIENTS:

- ¼ cup of apple cider vinegar
- 15 drops of peppermint essential oil
- 15 drops of lemon essential oil
- Water

INSTRUCTIONS:

- Mix vinegar and essential oil in a 16 oz. glass spray bottle.

- Fill the rest of the bottle with water.

- Shake well to combine all ingredients.

- Use the spray to sanitize your countertops, tiles, floors, and sinks.

Eucalyptus Essential Oil

Eucalyptus essential oil is a widely used natural remedy. Diffusing just a few drops into the air can help you kill germs, relieve a cough and clear sinuses. Using eucalyptus during flu seasons is especially recommended.

The antiseptic value of eucalyptus oil can be attributed to the component called eucalyptol also known as 1,8-cineole. This major constituent showed antimicrobial effects on bacteria that cause tuberculosis, drug-resistant bacteria causing staph infections, different viruses, and fungi, including Candida. Eucalyptus essential oil without a doubt one of the most versatile natural agents you can get your hands on.

TIPS FOR USE:

1. According to *The Scientific World Journal*, a strong minty, almost medicinal smell of eucalyptus repels house rats. To get rid of your rat problem, dilute 20 drops of eucalyptus oil in some water and spray the solution around your pantry and around small openings of your house. Keep in mind that eucalyptus essence may irritate your cat.

2. Add a couple of drops of eucalyptus essential oil to a cup of hot water. Use this solution to wipe down the corners where mold is prone to thrive.

3. Add 10-20 drops of eucalyptus oil to the washing cycle to eradicate dust mites from your linen, towels, and pillows.

4. Eucalyptus essential oil mixes well with peppermint, lavender, and lemon essential oils.

Clove Essential Oil

Clove essential oil is a natural antiseptic agent known for its spicy aroma. Its antibacterial and antifungal activity can be attributed to the compound called eugenol. Clove bud oil contains about 80 to 90% of eugenol. Research shows that E. coli, acne-causing *Staph aureus*, and pneumonia-causing *Pseudomonas aeruginosa* are especially sensitive to clove essence.

These antibacterial and antiviral properties of clove essential oil can help you disinfect your home, especially during cold and flu season. Airborne particles of essence will help you boost your immune system and give you a better chance at fighting bacteria and viruses.

TIPS FOR USE:

1. Diffuse clove essential oil into the air. Feel free to mix clove oil with other essential oils such as cinnamon bark, bergamot, lemon, grapefruit, lavender, and rosemary.

2. Use clove essential oil to kill mold in your bathroom. Dilute a ¼ teaspoon of clove oil in 1 liter of water. This solution can be sprayed on surfaces where mold tends to grow e.g. sinks, showers, outdoors and indoors walls etc. Let the spray sit on the area for at least an hour before removing it with a wet cloth or a brush. Make sure you use protective gloves when cleaning with clove. It is also recommended to do a test patch on the surface to make sure it does not get damaged.

Lemon Essential Oil

Lemon essential oil is a widely used natural remedy known for its disinfectant attributes. Limonene and b-pinene are two main components that give this volatile oil its antimicrobial properties. Feel free to use lemon essential oil around your home to get rid of harmful pathogens. The citrus lemon smell will enrich your kitchen and bathroom with a hint of freshness as well.

According to the scientific research, lemon essential oil is strong enough to inhibit bacteria *Listeria monocytogenes* inoculated in minced beef. The study suggests that lemon oil could be used as a natural agent for preventing food contamination.

Harmful bacteria, such as salmonella, E. coli, and *Staph aureus* can cause serious illnesses. Regular use of homemade lemon oil cleaners around the house will help you lower the chances of bacterial infections.

TIPS FOR USE:

1. Lemon essential oil can be used on stained clothes. Add a few drops of lemon oil on the stain. Immediately put the stained clothes in the washing machine.

2. If your hands are greasy from working on your car or bike, a few drops of lemon oil added to your soap can help you get rid of any greasy residue.

3. Lemon essential oil mixes well with eucalyptus, peppermint, geranium, and sandalwood.

4. Clean your windows and other glass surfaces with this lemon oil spray.

Lemon Oil Glass Cleaner

INGREDIENTS:

- 1 ½ cup of vinegar
- ½ cup distilled water
- 8 drops of lemon essential oil

INSTRUCTIONS:

- Mix all ingredients in a 16 oz. glass spray bottle.

- Wipe down your windows, mirrors, and shower doors with the solution.

Disinfect and polish your wooden floor and furniture with this natural lemon wood polish.

DR. BRADLEY SHAPERO, D.C.

Lemon Wood Polish

INGREDIENTS:

- ¼ cup vinegar
- ¼ cup olive oil
- 10 drops of lemon essential oil

INSTRUCTIONS:

- Combine all ingredients in a glass spray bottle.

- Using a microfiber cloth, wipe down wooden surfaces to give them shine.

- Use this natural polish every 3 months. Shake the bottle before each usage.

CHAPTER FIVE
PROTECT YOURSELF: THE FORCES WITHIN YOU

Scientists are discovering that while anger and hatred eat into our immune system, warm-heartedness and compassion are good for our health.

— Dalai Lama

The world has a different look when you peer through the lens of a microscope. Yael, whose code name in the Israel Defense Forces (IDF) was well known as "willing," was noticing some peculiar aspects of the SARS-Cov2 while sequencing the DNA. Her lab associate and handler Dany relayed the information to his team just prior to his sudden and questionable disappearance. The two had been working round the clock, in December 2019, decoding the virus and attempting to isolate its origin. Both had worked in BSL-4 labs from time to time although this project was assigned to a BSL-3 lab in an undisclosed location.

One week to the day that Dany went missing, Yael was confronted by three strangers who cautioned her to drop the project. Her expertise in immunology and bacteriology proved to be quite important as the world began to sink into a pool of fear and panic. The spread of the virus swiftly moved across borders and over the seas. Yael managed to secure two vials to work with as she went into hiding. In a secret lab, the research and testing continued. Through a complex network, her findings were deliberately leaked out to aid in the countermeasure. (PYGAS, 2014)

As Yael furthered her research, she discovered that she too had been exposed. However, what was puzzling was that she was only mildly symptomatic. If she had not been testing herself, she would not have known that her own body had begun rapidly making antibodies against the virus. Additionally, she was a big fan of citrus and noticed that naturally occurring Vitamin C along with Zinc was extremely important to her body developing the protection she now possessed. The body with its amazing defense, was set up to fight against foreign pathogens. Yael also discovered that the virus was not able to infect the host by just landing on the skin. Rather it had to be carried by droplets which either deposited in the nose, mouth, or possibly the eye.

The previous chapter dealt with external ways to protect your immune system, body and environment. Now let's dive inside your body and take a look at what you can do to greatly enhance the function of your immune system to provide the most protection.

There are essentially two systems in humans and higher life forms. These two immune systems have a variety of tools which are used that set up lines of defense to neutralize threats to your body. On a rudimentary level one system differentiates between self and non-self which is known as the Innate Immune System. The more highly evolved system is the Adaptive Immune System.

The adaptive immune system has in its arsenal several types of responses. The type of response that gets activated is determined by the Thymus gland. Depending on the challenge your body is facing your Thymus gland will activate particular white blood cells.

T cells (thymus gland) and B cells (bone marrow) derived are the major cellular components of the adaptive immune system. T cells are involved in cell-mediated immunity which means they seek out and neutralize invaders such as bacteria, viruses, and other foreign invaders. The B cells are primarily responsible for humoral immunity, which means antibodies. The function of T and B cells is to identify invaders and substances that are not part of the body known as "non-self" antigens.

An antigen is a substance, usually a protein that starts or causes an immune reaction. Once these cells identify an invader the body will generate a specific response that is tailored to eliminate the specific pathogen (viruses, bacteria, yeasts, molds, protozoans, etc.) or pathogen infected cells. When your immune system launches an attack to rid the body of a particular invader it will catalog the response in what is known as a memory cell. So, in the future if you are exposed again the response will be much quicker. The thymus gland writes up the battle plan for a particular pathogen and launches the response. The battle plan is then filed away so that it can be used again if you have a re-exposure.

The 2019-nCoV so far has shown several mutations or variations. About 70 per cent of the patient samples were from the more aggressive type of SARS-CoV-2, the virus that causes COVID-19. It is not uncommon for a virus to mutate however this one appears to mutate more rapidly. In theory you could contract one variant and then contract another from someone in your immediate circle of contacts who had a variant that mutated. This is why it is so imperative to maximize the efficiency and function of your immune system.

In my research, I came across Dr. Dan Dimkee, PhD who has some very compelling information to share and how the virus is affected by higher temperatures. There are also a number of research studies done which discuss the tolerance of a virus and particularly the coronavirus to various temperatures. I find this particularly relevant considering the body uses temperature as one of the lines of defense.

Your body temperature often rises because of an infection, when it does it's called a fever. Fevers that happen as the body's response to an infection rarely go over 106.2 (41.3 C). Such high temperatures are most commonly due to head trauma, heatstroke, poisoning or side effect of anesthesia.

It is important to keep in mind that fever in general is NOT dangerous. To damage the brain, our temperature would have to go over 107.6 F (42 C). Use the fever as a sign your body is sending you that some infection is going on and see if you can do something about it. Rest, nutrition high in vitamin C and other immune supporting supplements, fresh air, and light exercise can help your body's immune system to fight infection before it becomes serious.

Studies indicate that supporting the process with chiropractic care, homemade chicken soup with fresh vegetables and garlic are very helpful. See my simple recipe in the back of the book. In addition you may want to bundle up and allow the body to work through the fever and monitor so that it does not go over 105° F which it rarely does. However, do get some guidance from your health care professional or family chiropractor.

Fevers are caused by chemicals called pyrogens flowing in the bloodstream. Pyrogens make their way to the hypothalamus in the brain, which is in charge of regulating body temperature. When pyrogens bind to certain receptors in the hypothalamus, body temperature rises.

One common pyrogen is called Interleukin-1 (IL-1). IL-1 is produced by white blood cells called macrophages when they come into contact with certain bacteria and viruses. IL-1 has multiple purposes, one of which is to signal other white blood cells, called helper T cells, into action.

It is interesting to note that as problematic as this virus is it too has some weaknesses and is not as hearty as many might think. Viruses such as the SARS-CoV-2 thrive in colder temperatures and can survive near freezing. However, these same viruses are very susceptible to heat which is why they stay in the cooler areas of the body such as sinus cavities and lungs.

Dr. Lee Dimke points and numerous studies support that the coronavirus is easily killed in about 15 minutes at temperatures of 56°C or 133°F. By exposing a person to these temperatures and breathing in hot air the virus can be rendered incapacitated without harming the individual. In fact many deserts around the world reach temperatures of 110°F to 120°F and some over 130°F.

Many saunas range from 170°F to 195°F which is well above the necessary temperature. Saunas are fairly easy to find. Treatment would consist of breathing deeply for about 20 minutes in this type of a heated environment. This will kill most of the virus in the upper respiratory system. Repeat this treatment 2-3 times about an hour apart should kill the remaining viruses according to Dr. Dimke. Dr. Dimke suggests that using a hot blow dryer could also work but this method is controversial and stated as false from snopes. I suspect that using a blow dryer as suggested is challenging. One must attempt to raise the temperature to the desired level and sustain that for at least 20 minutes. The preferred and most controlled method is the use of a sauna. (Cold Arrest, 1994)

When dealing with this or any other pathogen it is vitally important to keep your immune system strong. Eat healthy nutrient dense foods, drink plenty of water, avoid alcohol, excessive amounts of refined carbohydrates and sweets. A healthy balanced diet, enough sleep, positive mental attitude, exercise and a proper functioning nerve system will maximize health. There are many types of nutrients which are needed for the body however, in this next section I focus on those particularly enhancing the immune system.

As was pointed out earlier the thymus gland is extremely important in the overall immune function. The process of identifying an invading pathogen and creating the antibodies takes about 7 days. The thymus can be greatly supported with bovine thymus gland.

Thymex: This is a product made from bovine thymus gland and promotes phagocytic and lymphatic activity. This is important with both bacterial and viral infections. This seeds and supports the gland which then produces antibodies.

Calcium Lactate: For the immune system to run effectively you must have calcium. However, it must be in the correct form. It must be able to get into the tissues of the body. Calcium Lactate which becomes Calcium *Bi*carbonate. NOT to be confused with calcium carbonate which is pretty useless in human physiology. Calcium bicarbonate is needed to help immune cells known as microphages and phagocytes move through the tissues in a process known as chemotaxis. Then calcium bicarbonate surrounds the infected cell signaling the immune cells to "kill this cell or invader and spare everyone else."

Calcium Lactate is converted to calcium bicarbonate in one quick step. This simple supplement is very important in prevention and recovering from an infection. Research has shown this to be very effective in preventing and recovering from various infectious agents such polio, bubonic plague and quite a few other viruses and bacteria.

There is a vast difference between naturally occurring vitamins and synthetic vitamins. Without going into too much detail on common difference is the shape of the molecule. Even though all the same pieces or molecules are present if they are arranged in a slightly different configuration it will not function the same way in the body.

Vitamin C: Naturally occurring vitamin C along with Vitamin A and P make a fantastic combination. This combination also helps with signaling and targeting pathogens for destruction. As well as assisting in tissue repair. Your immune system has some fascinating tools. Phagocytes are the cells that goggle up cells that are targeted for destruction, however, before this happens your body destroys these cells from the inside. Vitamin C is what is used in this process, not ascorbic acid, but whole vitamin C.

I often talk about balance in the body. Here is another interesting twist to the story. Your body creates and uses small packets of reactive oxygen species or "free radicals" to accomplish this task. If you consume too much antioxidant you could interfere with this process. The body creates these free radical packets and then shoots them into the cell which destroys the cell from the inside. Vitamin C is what is used to perform the mechanism of injecting the cells with the ROS packets. It is pretty well known that Vitamin C enhances immune function but not commonly known that ascorbic acid is actually NOT real naturally occurring vitamin C.

It appears that the medical community avoids in large part talking about dietary supplements, like vitamin C, as a part of a treatment plan for anything, much less COVID-19. We can already see the FDA red flags are popping up. I found two recent studies by the same authors, in two separate journals about vitamin C being used to shorten the length of ICU stays and the duration of mechanical ventilation.

Even mainstream media is reporting that Long Island, New York hospitals are using vitamin C for COVID-19 patients as part of an integrative treatment. Physicians there made the decision based on experimental treatments in Wuhan, China.

"The patients who received vitamin C did significantly better than those who did not get vitamin C," said Dr. Andrew G. Weber, a pulmonologist and critical-care specialist affiliated with two Northwell Health facilities on Long Island. "It helps a tremendous amount, but it is not highlighted because it's not a sexy drug," he told the New York Post. (See more details in Appendix 4)

Zinc: According to the American Society for Nutrition zinc is extremely important to the immune function. Zinc is an essential trace element that is crucial for growth, development, and the maintenance of immune function. It influences all organs and cell types, representing an integral component of approximately 10% of all the proteins in the human body (human proteome), and encompassing hundreds of key enzymes and transcription factors.

Zinc deficiency is strikingly common, affecting up to a quarter of the population in developing countries, but also affecting distinct populations in the developed world as a result of lifestyle, age, and disease-mediated factors. Consequently, zinc status is a critical factor that can influence antiviral immunity, particularly as zinc-deficient populations are often most at risk of acquiring viral infections such as HIV or hepatitis C virus. Zinc has become one of the most popular suggestions for reducing symptoms of coronavirus. Notably, an email written by a pathologist, Dr. James Robb, that recommends using zinc lozenges to ward off the virus, along with other tips, has gone viral. **For more information, check my websites:**

www.PremierHealthCareSC.com
www.DrBradShaperoOnline.com

For products links to our online store look in the back of the book under protocols.

HERBS ARE VERY POTENT FUNCTIONAL MODULATORS.

Andrographis: Andrographis paniculata is a bitter tasting annual plant, referred to as the "King of Bitters." It has white-purple flowers and it is native to Asia and India where it has been valued for centuries for its numerous medicinal benefits. is an excellent choice for acute immune challenges. Andrographis has shown to enhance lymphocyte function by enhancing the inflammatory mediator know has TNF- (Tumor Necrosis Factor alpha), enhances lymphocyte production, stimulates the immune response (cytokines), as well as enhances antibody response.

Echinacea: Taken along with natural vitamin C and Calcium Lactate, Echinacea is a fabulous broad-based immune support that has a great overall effect of boosting the immune system. Echinacea increases phagocyte activity, increases the dendritic cells which go out and get the information, stimulated NK (natural killer) cell production in the spleen, increases monocytes in the bone marrow, increases interferon production (interferon interferes or prevents viral replication). Although, Echinacea can do all these things it does not do them in a powerful fashion so it is best taken preventatively as well as in combination with the other items recommended.

Artemisinin: Also known as Sweet Wormwood, Artemisinin is found in China and Southeast Asia, particularly Vietnam. Tu Yu Yu, a Chinese medical researcher, received a Nobel Prize for her application of Artemisinin in Malaria cases, in 2015. The exact mechanism of action is still unknown but is thought to have something to do with destroying the pathogen using some sort of oxidative method. This herb has shown to be effective against Leishmania, Herpes, Giardia, just to name a few and many parasites as well. It is also well studied for its potent anti-cancer properties. The dosage is pulsed so that the liver does not build up detoxification enzymes against the herb which is counterproductive. Artemisinin interferes with the replication process of the infected cells which shuts down the replication of the virus.

Myrrh: This herb is still under much research. It seems to greatly accelerate the immune system. Specifically, in dendritic activity, which is the detection and identification of pathogens, along with increase Macrophage activity which engulfs the pathogen and destroys it.

Vironon: This is a proprietary blend of Thuja, St John's Wort, and Licorice. This is an amazing mixture combining the anti-viral activity of these three herbs making a potent blend. These seem to be affective with enveloped viruses such as theSARS-CoV-2. It seems to bind to the lipid envelope and render it inactive.

As of June 2020 there is no vaccine or drug that is a cure for SARS-CoV-2. The leading contender seems to be AstraZenteca and the University of Oxford. This vaccine is in the third phase of testing. However, there are some pharmaceuticals which have shown to have promising results. Keep in mind that all drugs have side effects. That being said let's explore some of these options. (See the Q&A section for more)

One option that is being explored are a set of pharmaceuticals know as anti-interleukin medication. These medications are used in conditions such as asthma, Crohn's disease, cancer and many others.

This type of intervention should be considered with great caution after many other tools have failed because this medication interferes with the body's own immune function and has many side effects.

Chloroquine phosphate: More commonly known for its use against Malaria, this has shown very promising results againstSARS-CoV-2. Chloroquine phosphate, an old drug for treatment of malaria, is shown to have apparent efficacy and acceptable safety against SARS-CoV-2 associated pneumonia in multiple clinical trials in different locations conducted in China. The drug is recommended to be included in the next version of the Guidelines for the Prevention, Diagnosis, and Treatment of Pneumonia Caused by SARS-CoV-2 issued by the National Health Commission of the People's Republic of China for treatment of SARS-CoV-2 infection in larger populations in the future. Science Direct published research which included six articles (one narrative letter, one in-vitro study, one editorial, expert consensus paper, two national guideline documents) and 23 ongoing clinical trials in China. This team of researchers concluded that Chloroquine seems to be effective in limiting the replication of SARS-CoV-2 (virus causing COVID-19) in vitro.

What I found very fascinating is why Chloroquine was effective. Chloroquine is an established antimalarial agent that has been recently tested in clinical trials for its anticancer activity. The favorable effect of chloroquine appears to be due to its ability to sensitize cancerous cells to chemotherapy, radiation therapy, and induce apoptosis. The present study investigated the interaction of zinc ions with chloroquine in a human ovarian cancer cell. Chloroquine enhanced zinc uptake. Fluorescent microscopic examination of intracellular zinc distribution demonstrated that free zinc ions are more concentrated in the lysosomes after addition of chloroquine, which is consistent with previous reports showing that chloroquine inhibits lysosome function.

The combination of chloroquine with zinc enhanced chloroquine's cytotoxicity and induced apoptosis. Thus chloroquine is a zinc ionophore, a property that may contribute to chloroquine's anticancer activity. At this point you may be thinking that this study relates to cancer cells and you are correct. However, keep in mind these two facts; it is well known that chloroquine (anti-malarial drug) is a zinc ionophore. Also, Chloroquine opens gates on the cell membrane, transports zinc into the cell, zinc shuts down the activity of RdRP and SARS-CoV-2 cannot replicate.

Take a look at what was done in South Korea. The death rates there were 1%. Compare that to China at 4%, Italy at 8%, Iran at 6% and the US at 2% (at the time of this writing, 3-18-2020). So, the South Koreans jumped on this immediately, have a good medical system, and have been doing research since the first minute of the crisis:but, it does cause one to think. Here is a paper from South Korea discussing the use of chloroquine (actually it discusses hydroxychloroquine which is an equivalent – from February 13, 2020)

Keep in mind that Chloroquine is not without its own set of side effects. Some have turned to tonic water (as a cheap over-the-counter diluted alternative) which has been diluted to attempt to avoid side effects and although serious side effects are unlikely, some of the more common side effects can still occur with Quinine in tonic water. If you do have a reaction, it may include:

- nausea
- stomach cramps
- diarrhea
- vomiting
- ringing in the ears
- confusion
- nervousness

Here are the protocols which are also found in the back of the book which give general guidelines to how these supplements should be taken in most cases. However, keep in mind individual health concerns and situations vary from person to person.

The following recommendations are products that I take and recommend to my patients to enhance the immune function and part of a first line of defense. They have proven quite effective in many types of conditions.

These products can be found on my own online store. Although each individual is unique and may require different amounts based on their health history and current health status as well as exposure, the first five products listed here would provide most people with a very strong overall protection and support for the immune system. These would typically be taken during times of increased exposure and when you feel your body needs some extra immune support.

For Maintenance and building up the immune function:

- Thymex: 4 daily
- Calcium Lactate: 3 - 2 times daily
- Cataplex ACP: 4 daily
- Zinc AG: 1 - 2 daily
- Echinacea Complex: 2 daily

For even more protection, consider adding the one or more of the following. If you feel you have a higher than average risk exposure and would like to add more protection than I suggest adding one or more of the following to the basic recommendation above.

- Andrographis Complex: 2 daily
- AdvaClear: 2 tablets daily.
- Sinuplex: 1 capsule twice daily.
- Artemisinin Complex: 1 daily
- Myrrh Forte: 1 daily
- Viranon: 2 daily
- Epimune Complex: 3 daily

During an active infection the dosage should be altered as suggested below which also varies from person to person.

- Thymex: 8 - 12 daily
- Calcium Lactate: In the acute phase you may need 4 – 6 per hour. Mixing in lemon water makes this easier.
- Cataplex ACP: 8 - 12 daily
- Andrographis Complex: 6 - 8 daily
- Zinc AG: 1 – 2 daily
- Echinacea Complex: liquid 5 ml 4 – 6 times daily

Add the following as needed depending on the severity

- AdvaClear: 2 tablets daily.
- Sinuplex: 1 capsule twice daily.
- Artemisinin Complex: 3 twice daily for 5 days (8 – 10 days off) repeat
- Myrrh Forte: 4 twice daily for 5 days (8 – 10 days off) repeat
- Viranon: 6 - 8 daily
- Epimune Complex: 8 - 12 daily

Supplements such as vitamins and minerals as well as many herbs support the body processes set up by the immune system to fight off invading pathogens. In an upcoming chapter we will take a look at how your immune system can be greatly enhanced by tuning up your nervous system.

The following recommendations are products that I take and recommend to my patients to enhance the immune function and part of a first line of defense. They have proven quite effective in many types of conditions.

These products can be found on my own online store:

Metagenics: http://premierhealthcare.metagenics.com/store

Practitioner Code: **PremierHealthCare**

Standard Process: https://www.standardprocess.com/
Patient-Direct/patient-registration

Patient Direct Code: **WQ45V2**

For maintenance and building up the immune function:

- Thymex: 4 daily
- Calcium Lactate: 3 – 2 times daily
- Cataplex ACP: 4 daily
- Zinc AG: 1 – 2 daily
- Echinacea Complex: 2 daily

For even more protection, consider adding the one or more of the following:

- Andrographis Complex: 2 daily
- AdvaClear: 2 tablets daily.
- Sinuplex: 1 capsule twice daily.
- Artemisinin Complex: 1 daily
- Myrrh Forte: 1 daily
- Viranon: 2 daily
- Epimune Complex: 3 daily

CHAPTER SIX
TAKE ACTION: IF YOU THINK YOU ARE INFECTED

*Begin to free yourself at once by doing all
that is possible with the means you have, and
as you proceed in this spirit the way will open
for you to do more.*

— Robert Collier

The flight from Thailand was uneventful. The airports were quieter than ever with hardly a line, including boarding. Randy's seat near the window was the only seat taken in the entire row. On the flight over, there were 478 passengers and this flight back there were 104 passengers. Going through customs was a breeze as he was the only one in line at the time. The ride back to his neighborhood was quiet. It was 3:30 pm and there were barely any cars out on the road. After making his way to the market and a few other errands, Randy noticed a slight soreness in his throat.

Quick to act, he made a solution of hydrogen peroxide and gargled. The soreness persisted so he continued to gargle every hour until the pain was gone. Just to be safe, he began taking some Echinacea, Vitamin C, and Zinc. After staying home for a couple days, a slight fever started. Within 5 days, Randy began to experience what he had only heard about. He went to his chiropractor which saw him after hours. The fever progressed to 103.5° and continued for about 6 hours before breaking. Randy continued with supporting the immune system and chiropractic care and was feeling better after about 6 days. He was smart to take swift action and support the body with important nutrition as well as chiropractic adjustments to support the nerve system response.

As is the case with many infections, the symptoms do not show up for a period of time after exposure. In the case of CoVid-19, you may not see symptoms for as long as 20 days or more. Although the estimations vary, it is typically agreed upon that the symptoms usually take anywhere from 2 to 14 days and 4 to 6 days is fairly typical.

The initial symptoms vary from no symptoms, mild symptoms to severe and in some cases death. The majority of the cases, over 80% are mild.

The initial symptoms most commonly experienced are the following:

- Fever
- Sore Throat
- Dry Cough
- Fatigue (often associated with general malaise or difficulty breathing)
- Shortness of breath
- Other symptoms can include:
- Aches
- Vomiting / Diarrhea

If any of the following symptoms are present immediate medical attention is recommended:

- Ongoing chest pain or pressure
- New confusion
- Difficulty waking up
- Bluish lips or face

When you have symptoms, they can be similar to a bad cold or the flu. Your history will be helpful in differentiating between the likely possibilities. Suspect COVID-19 if:

- You have a fever and breathing problems, and you've traveled to places where the virus has spread.
- You've been exposed to people who have it within the last 14 days.

If you or someone you know suspects exposure or the possibility of exposure, the following is recommended, in addition to the guidelines outlined in the previous chapter.

Gargle with an antiseptic mouth wash or an alcohol bases solution. If these are not available, you could use a clean alcohol such as vodka. Rinse and gargle and then spit out into the sink with running water.

1. Wash the externally exposed areas with warm water and soap.

2. You may also consider getting into a sauna for 20 minutes.

At the first sign of symptoms such as a sore throat do the above steps, see your chiropractor, and be sure to use nutritional support recommended.

As pointed out in the section regarding fevers, it is not uncommon to have a high fever. Symptoms will typically resolve within 10 to 14 days. If you or someone you know is sick or has tested positive for CoVid-19, certainly consult your health professional, in addition to the following:

1. Maintain as much as possible a positive mental attitude

2. Get plenty of rest (Typically 7 to 9 hours, which various)

3. Exercise your body daily (at a level that is consistent with how sick you are feeling – you may need to keep this very light and in more severe cases you may be bed ridden)

4. Eat a healthy well balanced diet (with a variety of vegetables –possibly soups which are easy to digest)

5. Drink plenty of water (typically half your weight in ounces)

6. Ensure your nervous system is free from interference with Chiropractic care

7. Supplement as needed (this varies from person to person)

- Thymex: 8 - 12 daily
- Calcium Lactate: In the acute phase you may need 4 – 6 per hour. Mixing in lemon water makes this easier.
- Cataplex ACP: 8 - 12 daily
- Andrographis Complex: 6 - 8 daily
- Zinc AG: 1 – 2 daily
- Echinacea Complex: liquid 5 ml 4 – 6 times daily

Add the following as needed depending on the severity
- AdvaClear: 2 tablets daily.
- Sinuplex: 1 capsule twice daily.
- Artemisinin Complex: 3 twice daily for 5 days (8 – 10 days off) repeat
- Myrrh Forte: 4 twice daily for 5 days (8 – 10 days off) repeat
- Viranon: 6 - 8 daily
- Epimune Complex: 8 - 12 daily

Many in the media seem to focus on age. Age alone is not as much of a factor as the health status of the individual. Just because it is common for a person of age to have more health problems does not mean that is the case for all older individuals. For example, let's applaud Italica Grondona who made a full recovery after spending more than 20 days in the hospital from COVID-19. Italica Grondona who came down with the dangerous virus and was admitted with mild heart failure in early March to San Martino hospital located in the northern Italian city of Genoa.

"She only had some mild coronavirus symptoms, so we tested her and she was positive, but we did very little, she recovered on her own," her doctor, Vera Sicbaldi, told the outlet.

"We nicknamed her 'Highlander'—the immortal," Sicbaldi said. "Italica represents a hope for all the elderly facing this pandemic."

Also noteworthy is that serological samples were taken, it is speculated that she is the first patient known that might have gone through the 'Spanish flu' since she was born in 1917 according to reporters from CNN. Additionally worth emphasizing is that she had VERY little intervention for the virus and recovered on her own according the attending physician.

CHAPTER SEVEN
CHIROPRACTIC CARE

*The doctor of the future will give no
medicine but will interest the patient in the
care of the human frame, in diet, and in the
cause and prevention of disease.*

— Thomas Edison

*The person who takes medicine must
recover twice, once from the disease
and once from the medicine.*

— William Osler, MD

Trish and John, long time patients, were so excited to depart from
the hectic schedules and unplug from the day to day hustle and
bustle. This was the first cruise they had ever been on. Even though
they had been married for nearly 6 years, they actually had not
officially had a honeymoon. They looked forward to seven days
on the water, a trip to be remembered. Little did they know that
the romantic bubble both had painted in their mind was about to
change abruptly. Two days out at sea had been filled with a nice
balance of fun activities and relaxation by the pool. The morning
of the third day, just after docking at the port, an announcement
came over the loud speaker. The broadcast started as most addresses
from the captain.

"Good morning folks, this is your captain speaking. We have just been alerted to a situation which is rapidly being contained, but at this time we ask that you not leave your cabin."

That was the entire announcement. It would be a full two hours before the follow up announcement arrived.

"Hello guests, this is your captain again. It looks like we have contained the situation, but are asking that you stay in your cabin at this time. We have confirmed that there is an outbreak of Coronavirus on board and have been instructed to head back to our destination of origin. We will be breaking up the dinner times and allowing guests to leave the cabins by section at this time."

Needless to say, this was not the romantic getaway Trish and John had intended. Once at home, the couple was escorted via a crew in hazmat attire to a remote section of a hotel which they would spend the next fourteen days in quarantine. Once the two were able to leave, their first stop before going home was to my office for chiropractic care. They were fortunate that they did not develop any symptoms and were able to at least be home and limit travel and interaction for a few weeks.

While at the office, both Trish and John learned important information about how chiropractic helped others in previous pandemic outbreaks.

Let's turn our attention now to a natural time proven treatment which improves immune function along with countless other benefits. Chiropractic treatment is used all over the world by millions.

Many have asked what role Chiropractic plays in the immune function. David L. Sackett, the modern founder of Evidence-Based Health provided clarity to the intention. An evidence-based practice, "...aims at integrating individual clinical expertise with the best available external clinical evidence from systemic research and patient values."

Every day, chiropractors make evidence-informed decisions with their patients. As a result, about a million times a day, safe, effective chiropractic care is provided world-wide.

Chiropractic is the study of health and what causes man to live.

— Dr. B.J. Palmer, Founder of the ICA

The conversation that the experts in public health have been promoting is to use every means available to support one's immune system during the pandemic. (Adequate sleep, good nutrition, frequent hand washing with soap, etc.) There are other factors to consider as well. For example, the stress every member of the public, first responders, and health care professionals are feeling as a result of the changes in their everyday lives from the global pandemic. This stress has created unprecedented levels of anxiety and fear. Scientific evidence has validated that long-term exposure to stress negatively effects the immune system.

The issue of anxiety and stress has become so prevalent that the Centers for Disease Control and Prevention (CDC) and the National Institutes of Health (NIH) have begun promoting information to the public. Consider the information on the CDC's website which says that stress during an infectious disease outbreak can include:

- Fear and worry about your own health and the health of your loved ones
- Changes in sleep or eating patterns
- Difficulty sleeping or concentrating, worsening of chronic health problems
- Increased use of alcohol, tobacco, or other drugs

One of the recommendations to support oneself through the stress is to 'take care of your body.' Vitalistic chiropractors address more than just the mechanics of the spine. Chiropractic supports the whole person.

As Dr. B.J. Palmer, writes, "While other professions are concerned with changing the environment to suit the weakened body, chiropractic is concerned with strengthening the body to suit the environment."

Considerable evidence has mounted to support active communication between the nervous system and the immune system. The nervous system, including the brain and the peripheral divisions can either stimulate or inhibit various activities of both the innate and adaptive immune systems. Conversely, the immune system, through the release of cytokines, can influence the activity of the nervous system. Several excellent reviews have addressed the subjects of nervous and immune system "cross-talk" in great detail. Very recently, however, several peptides, recognized initially for their neural or neuroendocrine signaling functions have been shown to exhibit potent antimicrobial activity. This discovery signals the possibility that the nervous system, through utilization of these peptides, has the capacity to deliver anti-infective agents directly to innervated sites localized with great specificity and delivered rapidly. The nervous and neuroendocrine systems, in principle, have the potential to serve a direct immune function.

There are many studies that support the benefits of chiropractic care on the immune function. Here are some of those studies:

Neuroimmunomodulation and a Possible Correlation with Musculoskeletal System Function From 1989 states, "There is an increasing body of evidence that the nervous system is capable of modulating the immune response. Receptors for neuromodulators and neurohormones have been found on human T lymphocytes."

A Literature Review sought to determine the effects of spinal manipulation on biochemical markers in humans and establish the level of evidence for changes in biochemical biomarkers. Spinal Manipulation (SM), defined as a high-velocity, low amplitude thrust technique. Among the outcome measured sought were neuropeptides (neurotensin, oxytocin, SP) (2) inflammatory (TNF, IL) and (3) endocrine (cortisol, epinephrine, nor-epinephrine, luteinizing hormone) biomarkers from any body fluids (blood/urine/saliva). After removal of duplications, 1217 citations were screened. That was culled down to 96 abstracts screened, 45 full-text articles were assessed for eligibility. And a total of 8 trials included in the review. The conclusion after the review was that a moderate level of evidence existed in the eight studies which found that spinal manipulation influences various biomarkers typically identified as ones not only involved in pain perception/modulation but also play an important role in inflammation, tissue healing and immune response.

The outcomes of the study, Spinal Manipulation effect on interleukin-2 production, included a statistically significant increase in the production of IL-2 in both of the arms of the study in which patients received spinal manipulation relative to baseline and to the control group at 20 minutes post adjustment.

Dr. Pero, Ph.D. measured the immune systems of people under chiropractic care as compared to those in the general population and those with cancer and other serious diseases. In his initial three-year study of 107 individuals who had been under chiropractic care for five years or more, the chiropractic patients were found to have a 200% greater immune competence than people who had not received chiropractic care, and 400% greater immune competence than people with cancer and other serious diseases. The immune system superiority of those under chiropractic care did not diminish with age. Dr. Pero stated: When applied in a clinical framework, I have never seen a group other than this chiropractic group to experience a 200% increase over the normal patients. This is why it is so dramatically important. We have never seen such a positive improvement in a group Pero R. "Medical Researcher Excited by CBSRF Project Results."The Chiropractic Journal, August 1989; 32.

THE 1918 INFLUENZA HISTORY

Chiropractors are typically taught the history of chiropractic including the account prepared by Wayne R. Rhodes, DC in writing about the history of chiropractic in the state of Texas. While this is not a scientific paper, it was published by Dr. Rhodes' peers in the Texas Chiropractic Association.

"The 1917 - 1918 influenza epidemic swept silently across the world bringing death and fear to homes in every land. Disease and pestilence, especially the epidemics, are little understood even now and many of the factors that spread them are still mysterious shadows, but in 1917-1918 almost nothing was known about prevention, protection, treatment or cure of influenza. The whole world stood at its mercy, or lack of it."

He continues, "Chiropractors got fantastic results from influenza patients..." The statistics speak for themselves: In 1918, a time when there were no validated treatments for flu, the epidemic killed millions world-wide.

Data Provided from the 1918 Spanish Flu Comparing Treatment/Death Numbers				
Location	Patients Treated by Medical Doctors (MDs)	Deaths in Medical Patients	Number of Patients Treated by Doctors of Chiropractic (DCs)	Deaths in Chiropractic Patients
Davenport, Iowa	4,953	274	1,635	1
State of Iowa	93,590	6,116 (1 in 15 deaths)	(Excluding Davenport) – 4,735	6
State of Oklahoma			3,490	7
	In Oklahoma, after medical doctors gave up 233 patients as lost, chiropractors were called in with 208 survivors and 25 deaths			
Nationally			46394	54
New York City Influenza	For every 10,0000	950	For every 10,000	25
New York City Pneumonia	For every 10,000	6400	For every 10,000	100

Chiropractic was also used in France. Dr. S.T. McMurrain (DC) provided care in the influenza ward of Base Hospital No. 84 in Perigau. The medical officer in charge during the outbreak sent all influenza patients for chiropractic adjustments. The outcomes were so impressive that Dr. McMurrain would be commissioned in the Sanitary Corps.

CONCLUSION

Chiropractic is a health care discipline which emphasizes the inherent recuperative power of the body to heal itself without the use of drugs or surgery. The practice of chiropractic focuses on the relationship between structure (primarily the spine) and function (as coordinated by the nervous system) and how that relationship affects the preservation and restoration of health. It is founded upon the principle that the body's innate recuperative power is affected by and integrated through the nervous system.

The current global health crisis surrounding the COVID-19 Pandemic has resulted in changes in our everyday lives and has created increased levels of stress and anxiety, and fear. Scientific evidence has validated that long-term exposure to stress negatively effects the immune system.

As an essential health care provider, I am in a unique position to assist my patients during this time of heightened stress. Although there are no clinical trials to substantiate a direct causal relationship between the chiropractic adjustment and increased protection from the SARS-CoV-2 virus, there is a growing body of evidence that there is a relationship between the nervous system and the immune system. As a service to patients in my community and around the world, I am committed to continue to look for and make available a library of relevant scientific evidence.

Taking into consideration the above information, I have prepared some recommendations for prevention as well as if you feel you have the disease.

Here is the fundamental guideline which I feel will give you the best protection based on the scientific evidence presented thus far:

- Maintain a positive mental attitude.
- Get plenty of rest. (Typically, 7 to 9 hours, which various)
- Exercise your body daily.
- Eat a healthy well-balanced diet with a variety of vegetables.
- Drink plenty of water, typically half your weight in ounces.
- Ensure your nervous system if free from interference with Chiropractic care
- Use supplement as needed (this varies from person to person)

CHAPTER EIGHT
THINK AHEAD: LOOK AROUND THE CORNER

*The great successful men of the world have
used their imaginations... they think ahead and
create their mental picture, and the go to work
materializing that picture in all its details, filling in
here, adding a little there, altering this a bit and
that a bit, but steadily building / steadily building.*

— Robert Collier (American motivational author, 1885-1950)

I have a friend who lives in the desert. After the outbreak, Tim was telling me that he was very prepared for just about anything. Tim listed off about 20 items that he had purchased the month before. Things like a generator, water filtration unit, first aid supplies etc. In our conversation on preparation, I asked him how he settled on certain brands. Tim seemed to have done his research

I asked what I thought was a pretty basic question. "When you tested out these items, did they perform as expected, and how long did it take you to deploy these things?"

There was a long pause before he admitted most of the items were still in the box. At which point, he realized that if he had a tool for any emergency situations it was vital to learn to use them before a situation breaks out.

You do not want to figure out how to assemble something that is needed during an emergency, just as you wouldn't want to figure out how to apply a tourniquet if someone was bleeding in front of you.

Tim had an important "Ah-ha" moment after that conversation. Part of preparation is staying healthy and training with the equipment you have so that you can use what you need when you need it without delay.

The best time to plan is before something happens, as the age-old adage states, "An ounce of prevention is worth a pound of cure." In the months ahead, I have no doubt we will get through this and look back and wonder how we got here?"

Take a moment and assess where you are. What type of preparation do you need to get you and those you care about ready for the next situation so you are not caught off guard? Prepare a list of what you need and the actions you can take to systematically work through the list. Avoid panicking and spending huge amounts of money to prepare. Simply get the basics to start and then add to it as time goes on.

Keep in mind that the way you prepare depends on the type of likely situations you will encounter and the environment where you live. Being near the ocean will be different than if you lived in the mountains. Preparing for a power outage is different than preparing for a hurricane or an earthquake. And these are vastly different than preparing for an unthinkable active shooter situation.

The military uses a system of preparedness known as the Force Protection Condition (FPcon) that identifies five levels of readiness to respond to a threat. Delta: Terrorist action against a specific location imminent. Charlie: Terrorist targeting against personnel and facilities is imminent. Bravo: Predictable terrorist threat activity exist. Alpha: Possible terrorist activity. Normal: Routine security posture. Whenever there is a situation such as a natural disaster or in this case the Covid-19 the intensity of the situation can open the door for terrorist opportunity. So this level also gives one perspective as to the level of perceived threat there is based on our military posturing.

Currently the local military base in Southern California where I live and practice is at FPcon bravo, which is the third level out of five. Authorities indicate that we may upgrade that to the next level which means that a terrorist threat is likely. The local health authorities are keeping things shut down. Despite the situation, it is important that communities work together to help those affected by the disease as well as the ripple effect from the closures and the disruption of day to day activities including work for many people.

The best investment you can ever make is the investment in yourself. Take a little time each day or each week to improve or maintain your health and skills. Even if you have trained in the past and do not periodically use those skills, they may not be there when you need them most, unless you train periodically. Obtaining and maintaining optimum health and wellbeing is a lifelong endeavor.

Invest in your physical, mental, and spiritual health. When you feel balanced at the level you are at, reach out and pull someone else up. The way we improve the world around us is by helping those around us and encouraging them to help others as well. For now we are all on the same boat, the S.S. Planet Earth hurling through space. The future truly does lie in our hands, in our ability to find creative healthy solutions to the situations we face. We can learn from yesterday as we busy ourselves in creating habits today to shape a future we can be proud of.

If you found this information helpful, recommend this book to a friend or family member. You can create your own ripple effect in this world by performing acts of kindness like a simple smile to a stranger, a helping hand to a neighbor, or offering a cup of tea or coffee to a friend. Do something to better someone else's experience today. That ripple may gain enough momentum that it will return as a wave that lifts you and the world up.

Blessings to you and yours and may you have a healthier tomorrow.

QUESTIONS & ANSWERS

This book is not intended as a substitute for the medical advice of physicians. The reader should regularly consult a physician in matters relating to his/her health and particularly with respect to any symptoms that may require diagnosis or medical attention.

The information presented in the pages of this book is offered for educational and informational purposes only, and should not be construed as personal medical advice.

You have not become a patient of Dr. Shapero by reading these pages, and you should consult with your personal physician/care giver regarding your own medical care.

Q. What is CoVid-19?

A. The CoVid-19 is, as of December 2019, the disease caused by, SARS-CoV-2, the latest of a family of coronaviruses which is airborne and can infect humans causing respiratory disease. Keep in mind that there are two types of airborne pathogens. This type must be carried on droplets and does not float around.

Elderly and high-risk people should take precautions to avoid even moderately populated areas.

Q. What are the symptoms of CoVid-19?

A. The common symptoms range from sore throat, fever and shortness of breath, even loss of taste and smell to more severe such as gastrointestinal problems, work of breathing, and in severe cases multi system failure.

If you are in the higher risk or elderly category, take the necessary steps to enhance your immune system.

A study conducted by the highly respected medical journal *The Lancet* found the following prevalence of symptoms:

- fever -experienced by 83% of patients
- cough -82%
- bilateral pneumonia -75%
- shortness of breath -31%
- acute respiratory distress syndrome -17%
- muscle ache -11%
- confusion -9%
- headache-8%
- sore throat-5%
- rhinorrhea-4%
- chest pain-2%
- diarrhea-2%
- nausea and vomiting-1%

Q. What is the test for CoVid-19?

A. The quick screening is taking of the temperature. However, there are currently two conformational tests which are similar. One is known as reverse-transcriptase polymerase chain reaction, or RT-PCR, to rapidly identify the presence of viral RNA in swabs from the noses of potentially infected people. The other is known as Nucleic Acid Amplification (NAA) done with a swab sample from the nasal or mouth area.

Q. How long can the virus live outside the body?

A. Some studies have also shown the stability of the virus typically will only live for about 3 hours airborne.

The study published by the New England Journal of Medicine examined the stability of the coronavirus strain on various materials, such as plastic, stainless steel and cardboard.

The study found that SARS-CoV-2 was more stable on plastic and stainless steel than on copper and cardboard. A viable virus was detected on those surfaces for up to 72 hours after application.

The virus was only viable for four hours on copper and for 24 hours on cardboard.

The temperature, the humidity, and whether the surface is smooth or porous can all affect how long the virus survives.

In most cases, when you use the basic hygienic practices of washing your hands with soap and warm water along with a healthy diet, you will greatly reduce your likelihood of infection.

Q. When should I call my doctor?

A. If you develop any of the following symptoms, stay home and contact your healthcare provider:

- cough
- fever
- body aches
- shortness of breath
- fatigue

The elderly and those with chronic medical conditions can be at increased risk when it comes to infection by the SARS-CoV-2. These individuals should take greater precautions to protect themselves. At the first sign of a sore throat gargle with hydrogen peroxide and warm water. (two ounces of Hydrogen Peroxide to 6 or 8 ounces of warm water)

Q. How can you tell the difference between the coronavirus, the common cold, the flu, and hay fever or other allergies

A. Even though there is a high concern about the 2019 novel coronavirus, it is still not difficult to catch a common cold, the flu, or experience other seasonal allergies such as hay fever. Keep in mind allergies and hay fever are not contagious. Because the symptoms of CoViD-19 disease can appear similar to the symptoms of the common cold, flu, and even seasonal allergies, knowing the differences in symptoms for each of these conditions can be beneficial and reduce unneeded worry and anxiety. However, one important factor in differentiating all the others from CoVid-19 is the health and travel history.

The tips and valuable information provided in this book will also help you reduce your exposure risk to the nCoVid-19, as well as other viruses and bacteria.

Q. What is the best protection against CoVid-19?

A. Your best protection is to avoid exposure and enhance your immune system. Those who are higher risk such as elderly and those with underlying health challenges should avoid high traffic times at the store. As well as utilize chiropractic care.

Q. What is the best source of information regarding SARS-CoV-2 and CoVid-19?

A. There are a variety of sources such as the World Health Organization, Centers for Disease Control, National Institute of Health, and peer reviewed studies.

Q. Why are people getting Covid-19 again? How does that relate to herd immunity?

A. Currently I am aware of eight different strains. Roughly 70% of the cases tested can be attributed to the two most viral strains. Typically immunity to one strain does not necessarily give you immunity to another. Researchers have stated that it appears the virus is mutating to less viral forms and is mutating relatively slowly. If you are exposed to another strain then you would need to develop immunity to that particular strain. Herd immunity would apply for a particular strain.

Q. **How likely will a timely vaccine be developed and how safe would it be.**

A. Regardless of your position on vaccines there are many that are under development. The timeline of a vaccine varies greatly despite what the media or politicians say a vaccine typically takes about 12 to 18 months to develop. (Dresden, 2020) The safety of this vaccine will be unknown for now. Any vaccine holds with it inherent risks which include permanent damage to the individual and death. I encourage you to be fully informed by reputable sources before submitting to an injectable substance. In an effort to minimize any anti-vaccine resistance the side effects of the vaccines being developed have been censored. Symptoms such as fever, malaise and nausea on the milder side. About 10% of the volunteers had fevers; other symptoms included skin rashes, fatigue etc. In fact what has been down played is that 80% of the volunteers of the vaccine trials experience headaches, chills and fatigue some had much worse symptoms. The fact that adverse reactions are being glossed over does not help confidence of the vaccines usage. If you or someone you know has an adverse reaction to a vaccine you should report it to the Vaccine Adverse Event Reporting System. https://vaers.hhs.gov/

PROTOCOLS
DR SHAPERO'S HOMEMADE CHICKEN SOUP:

There are many wonderful memories of my mother's cooking and one of the favorites was mom's chicken soup. Make sure to add lots of the secret ingredient.

In a large pot put in about 2 cups of water.
Dice the following as desired:

1. Potatoes
2. Carrots
3. Onions
4. Celery

Add minced garlic and white pepper. Use one carton of chicken broth as desired and simmer.

Add chicken and Matzo balls.

Oh, and of course the secret ingredient. Add some Love. Powerful enhancing agent.

That's it. This is a simple and easy to cook recipe.

Immune Boosting Smoothies

Smoothies are a great way to pack in lots of nutrient dense foods into a small meal. It's fast, simple and easy clean up. I have dozens of recipes and try out new combinations regularly. I recommend starting out with a few basic recipes that you like and have fun adding a few extras to the basic recipe. Have fun, be creative and take a moment to enjoy the flavors.

A few tips:

I suggest using fresh over frozen however if you want it to be more chilled then use frozen fruit. I just buy fresh and then freeze a small container.

1. My preference is to keep it real. You may substitute eggs for a cold pressed protein powder. Also, 1 egg is about 7 ½ grams of protein so adjust the eggs to desired protein level.
2. When adding fats use high quality oil.
3. The process is pretty simple whichever recipe you use which is to place all ingredients in a high-speed blender, and blend to the desired consistency. If you aren't using frozen blueberries, you can add a small handful of ice to cool it down.

Acai Green

Ingredients

- 1 egg
- 1/4 – 1/2 avocado
- 1 tbsp. chia seeds
- handful of spinach (about a ½ to ¾ cup)
- 1 tbsp. acai powder
- 1/4 cup organic fresh wild blueberries
- 1 cups unsweetened almond milk

Coconut Turmeric Cream

Ingredients

- 1 egg
- About a quarter cup of shaved coconut.
- 1 tbsp. coconut butter or MCT oil
- 2 tbsp. Acacia Fiber
- 1 cup unsweetened almond milk
- 1 tbsp. Turmeric Powder
- 1/4 cup fresh raspberries
- Optional – half a banana

Spa Smoothie

Ingredients

- 1 egg
- 1/4 avocado
- 1 to 2 tbsp. chia seeds
- juice of 1 lemon
- handful of spinach (about a ½ to ¾ cup)
- 1 small Persian cucumber
- 1/4 cup fresh mint leaves
- 1 cup unsweetened nut milk

Online Stores:
Metagenics: http://premierhealthcare.metagenics.com/store

Practitioner Code: **PremierHealthCare**

Standard Process: https://www.standardprocess.com/
Patient-Direct/patient-registration

Patient Direct Code: **WQ45V2**

The summary of maintaining optimum immune function.

1. Maintain a positive mental attitude.
2. Get plenty of rest (Typically 7 to 9 hours, which varies)
3. Exercise your body daily (at a level that is consistent with how sick you are feeling – you may need to keep this very light and in more severe cases you may be bed ridden)
4. Eat a healthy well balanced diet with fresh fruits and vegetables. (with a variety of vegetables –possibly soups which are easy to digest)
5. Drink plenty of clean water (typically half your weight in ounces)
6. Ensure your nervous system is free from interference with Chiropractic care
7. Supplement as needed (this varies from person to person)

    a. Thymex: 4 daily

    b. Calcium Lactate: 3 – 2 times daily

    c. Cataplex ACP: 4 daily

    d. Zinc AG: 1 – 2 daily

    e. Echinacea Complex: 2 daily

For even more protection, consider adding the one or more of the following:

    f. Andrographis Complex: 2 daily

    g. AdvaClear: 2 tablets daily.

    h. Sinuplex: 1 capsule twice daily.

    i. Artemisinin Complex: 1 daily

CORONAVIRUS

Modify the above protocol if you become infected:

a. Thymex: 8 - 12 daily

b. Calcium Lactate: In the acute phase you may need 4 - 6 per hour. Mixing in lemon water makes this easier.

c. Cataplex ACP: 8 - 12 daily

d. Andrographis Complex: 6 - 8 daily

e. Zinc AG: 1 - 2 daily

f. Echinacea Complex: liquid 5 ml 4 - 6 times daily

Add the following as needed depending on the severity

g. AdvaClear: 2 tablets daily.

h. Sinuplex: 1 capsule twice daily.

i. Artemisinin Complex: 3 twice daily for 5 days (8 - 10 days off) repeat

j. Myrrh Forte: 4 twice daily for 5 days (8 - 10 days off) repeat

k. Viranon: 6 - 8 daily

l. Epimune Complex: 8 - 12 daily

Travel or High Risk Exposure
If you need to travel or work in high risk areas take these simple precautions. These can be purchased in a kit or separately.

Use prudent hygiene habits as washing hands and use gloves when needed. Protective eye wear should be considered if you are in an area that is contaminated.

1. N95 Mask
2. Stress and Adrenal Support

3. Sleep and Rest Support
4. Herbal Throat Spray Phytosynergist® (This can also be swabbed in the nose as needed)
5. Thymex: 2 - 4 daily
6. Zinc AG: 1 daily

Elderly, High Risk and Multiple System Illnesses: If you are elderly, considered high health risk or have multiple system illnesses consider the following guidelines to minimize your exposure.

Minimize the circle of people you interact with from day to day.

1. Avoid high contact areas such as public gatherings and social events, travel should be avoided or limited to local areas.
2. Engage in activities which reduce stress and elevate your mood or emotion. Music, comedy, yoga, exercise and creative activities are good for this.
3. Use prudent hygiene habits as washing hands and use gloves when needed. Protective eye wear should be considered if you are in an area that is contaminated.
4. N95 Mask as needed when you are in higher contact areas
5. Stress and Adrenal Support
6. Sleep and Rest Support
7. Herbal Throat Spray Phytosynergist® (This can also be swabbed in the nose as needed)
8. Thymex: 3 – 4 daily
9. Calcium Lactate: 3 - 2 times daily
10. Cataplex ACP: 3 – 4 daily
11. Zinc AG: 1 daily
12. Echinacea Complex: 2 daily
13. Additional support may be needed depending on your circumstances, health status and exposure.

APPENDIX A

This virus is of the Genus Betacoronavirus, the species type is Murine Corona virus. The coronavirus family is divided into four groups (genera): alpha, beta, gamma, and delta. There are various subtypes which are identified by an alpha numeric combination such as HKU1, 229E, OC43, etc.

This is a new group of virus which at the time included infectious bronchitis from chickens, hepatitis virus from mice, and a gastrointestinal virus of swine.

Within the large family of virus, which is typically confined to animals, there have been seven identified to date that are Zoonotic, meaning they are capable of infecting humans. In fact, according to the CDC, zoonotic infection is very common with estimations of nearly 60% of human infections originally came from animals. SARS-CoV (Severe Acute Respiratory Syndrome Coronavirus) quickly spread around the world affecting 26 countries in 2003 was associated with bats. Palm civets and a racoon dog are thought to have acted as possible intermediaries for the virus which is thought to have originated from bats in Southern China where the disease claimed to have originated. SARS-CoV presents with symptoms similar to the Influenza which at the time infected over 8000 people and a death toll of nearly 800. Health officials scrambled to contain the outbreak and as far as we know this was self-limiting with no new cases identified since 2004. (Kahn & McIntosh, 2005)

In 2012 MERS-CoV (Middle East Respiratory Syndrome Coronavirus Virus) came onto the scene, first identified in Saudi Arabia. The dromedary camel is credited as being the main reservoir host for this infection. Although, MERS does not seem to be easily transmitted except through close contact human to human transmission has accounted for most of the infected cases. The vast majority of the cases have been seen in Saudia Arabia, United Arab Emeritus, and the Republic of Korea.

The symptoms range from asymptomatic and mild to death. Including gastrointestinal symptoms, pneumonia, and due to the intensity can complicate other illnesses such as kidney, liver, or other problems affecting the respiratory system.

Although, the reported mortality rate of MERS-CoV is 35% which is quite high, this number is very likely quite inflated due to the number of mild cases and asymptomatic cases which never actually got counted. The mortality numbers were only counted among the laboratory confirmed cases according to sources from WHO.

The origin of this may have been bats many years ago with the intermediary in our current time being the dromedary camel. 80% of the cases have been seen in Saudi Arabia with cases also appearing in Algeria, Austria, Bahrain, China, Egypt, France, Germany, Greece, Islamic Republic of Iran, Italy, Jordan, Kuwait, Lebanon, Malaysia, the Netherlands, Oman, Philippines, Qatar, Republic of Korea, Kingdom of Saudi Arabia, Thailand, Tunisia, Turkey, United Arab Emirates, United Kingdom, United States, and Yemen, since 2012.

Mid-summer of 2019 GeneOne Life Science released that it had completed Phase I of its testing on a vaccine for MERS. The GLS-5300 MERS CoV vaccine was tested on 75 military personnel at the Walter Reed Army Institute of Research (WRAIR) Clinical Trials Center in the first in-person test. No major reactions have been reported. However, keep in mind that this test was on young healthy individuals. The study is moving forward to a second Phase I/IIa trial in South Korea and a Phase II study in the Middle East.

In an effort to give some context to the current situation and give a small picture of the evolution of how the 2019-nCoV came onto the scene we have explored the previous outbreaks of CoV in our recent history. It was first known as SARS-CoV2 and has many names Severe Acute Respiratory Syndrome Coronavirus 2, COVID-19, Novel Coronavirus, 2019-nCoV, 2019 Novel Coronavirus, and Novel 2019 Coronavirus currently and now commonly called CoVid-19 although more precisely the virus is known as SARS-CoV-2 and the disease is CoVid-19. This novel coronavirus appeared on the scene in December 2019, in the city of Wuhan, China.

APPENDIX B

There have been claims that virology labs around the world have run a genomic analysis of the 2019 coronavirus giving indication that the coronavirus may have been engineered by human scientists. The proof is in the virus itself: The tools for genetic insertion are still present as remnants in the genetic code. Since these unique gene sequences don't occur by random chance, they is proof that this virus was likely engineered by scientists in a lab.

The WHO and CDC may be covering up this inconvenient fact in order to protect communist China and its biological weapons program, since no government wants the public to know the full truth about how frequently government-run labs experience outbreaks. Decades ago, for example, the U.S. Army ran an Ebola bioweapons lab in the United States where a monkey infected one of the scientists there. The strain turned out to be infectious only in monkeys, not humans, so the world dodged a bullet, but the U.S. Army "nuked" the entire facility with chemical bombs, killing all the monkeys and wiping out any last remnant of the virus on U.S. soil.

You can read the full details of that incident in the book *The Hot Zone* by Richard Preston. I've also seen it covered at NaturalNews. com, where this book description is reprinted:

In 1989, Reston, VA—one of the most famous U.S. planned communities located about 10 miles from Washington DC— stood at the epicenter of a potential biological disaster. This well-known story was narrated by Richard Preston in a bone chilling account related to the recognition and containment of a devastating tropical filovirus at a monkey facility—the Reston Primate Quarantine Unit.

That outbreak occurred because Ebola was found to be *spreading through the air ducts*, confirming that Ebola can spread through the air. This simple fact was vigorously covered up by the entire medical establishment during the Ebola scare in the United States many years later, where the CDC transported an infected patient to a hospital in Dallas, subsequently infecting a nurse who was treated with highly toxic chemicals. They caused permanent kidney damage. She later sued the hospital for the damage she suffered.

This incident is relevant because we know that virology labs routinely experience contamination lapses. Even here in the United States when studying deadly viruses we have seen facilities fail to contain these substances. Biological labs are graded by safety level. Level four is the highest level. One of China's top virology labs which is a P4 lab known as the Wuhan Institute of Virology has been on the suspect list due to its proximity to ground zero. This may or may not be well founded. China's BSL-4 labs have had multiple accidental releases of SARS strains.

The Washington Times quoted former Israeli intelligence officer Dany Shoham as claiming The Wuhan Institute of Virology is part of a secret biological weapons program.

"Certain laboratories in the institute have probably been engaged, in terms of research and development, in Chinese (biological weapons), at least collaterally, yet not as a principal facility," he asserted without corroborating evidence.

Mr. Shoham says he was a Mossad lieutenant colonel specialist in biological and chemical warfare. But so far he's the only apparent expert to make such a link.

However, Vipin Narang, MIT security studies professor warns, "There is no evidence that it was a bioweapon, and any claims that it is willfully spreads misinformation and is incredibly irresponsible."

On the other hand some still assert that in light of the type of testing and research which goes on in this facility and some evidence that this may have been an engineered strain that was either used in bioweapons research or vaccine experiments.

It was puzzling to me to find out that in most states that if the cause of death is suspected but no confirmed diagnosis is made it can be attributed to Covid-19. In a report reviewing cause of death it was determined that as much as 88% of deaths involving Covid-19 deaths were not caused by Covid-19. Why? Good question. Perhaps it has something to do with the fact that Medicare pays hospitals $13,000 for admissions diagnosed with Covid-19 and the number goes up to $39,000 if that person is put on a ventilator. I actually don't think the two are directly related but I do think there are some interesting questions that certainly warrant a clear answer.

My position on vaccines is that the receiver is fully informed and gives consent to the procedure, that each individual has a right to choose for themselves. The controversy of vaccines has been argued among the health care community for some time. Due to the amount of vaccine injuries the US Government formed the National Childhood Vaccine Injury Act of 1986 by Ronald Regan. This in effect shifted the liability of vaccines from the manufacturer to you the tax payer. I simply urge the reader to look closely with an open mind into the research and data available regarding this topic and the motives that in some instances are far from humanitarian.

A recent example is the use of HCG in a tetanus vaccine used in Kenya. The adjuvant is known to cause sterilization. Why was this included in a tetanus vaccine? Currently polio vaccine is responsible for most of the polio found in the world today. My point in bringing this up is that there are currently talks about having markers in the current Covid-19 vaccine. Let's keep in mind the Holocaust and those who were marked. *"The invisible "tattoo" accompanying the vaccine is a pattern made up of minuscule quantum dots—tiny semi-conducting crystals that reflect light—that glows under infrared light. The pattern—and vaccine—gets delivered into the skin using hi-tech dissolvable microneedles made of a mixture of polymers and sugar."*

There has been much talk around the globe of using RFID (Radio Frequency Identification) and Micro chip implants as well as Quantum Dots. These are implanted identification tools. I would encourage you to look into both of these things so that you are fully aware of what is happening in the way of your privacy and tracking.

In Late May 2020 reports began to build from the CDC as well as other sources that the testing for Covid-19 is unreliable. It is no surprise that the general public is confused about the real picture of what is going on here. Testing is showing both false positive and false negative results. The actual numbers reported are based on both symptom profiles and testing. When the data source is unreliable the entire statistical assessment becomes inaccurate. In light of the fact that this virus is like no other we have seen on the Corona virus family and there is reason to have some reasonable caution as to handling it. Keep in mind that the research is still done on a lower level biological lab. To complicate matters there seem to be several underlying agendas which have altered the true picture and created unreasonable fear in the general public.

We can be sure of one thing and, this is my opinion, that although we may not actually get to the full truth, I suspect it may take months to uncover most of the actual facts.

It may be interesting to note although perhaps unrelated that there has been a large spike in the number of sealed indictments being issued in the months leading up to this situation. An indictment is a formal accusation of a felony, issued by a grand jury based upon a proposed charge, witnesses' testimony and other evidence presented by the public prosecutor (District Attorney).

A sealed indictment is an indictment that is sealed so that it stays non-public until it is unsealed. This can be done for a number of reasons. It may be unsealed, for example, once the named person is arrested.

From 10/30/2017 to 09/30/19, 124,558 sealed indictments are set up from United States Federal District Criminal Courts. A monthly average of almost 6,000 new indictments in 2019, an increase of 5,000 acts per month on average compared to 2018 which only counted 1,000 to 2,000 sealed indictments per month!

Some have claimed that the concentration of indictments and cases of CoVid-19 seem to have some correlation. I will leave that and some of the other loose ends above for you to decide. Perhaps more compelling evidence will present itself in the months ahead.

Either way there are quite a number of questions and facts that do not seem to make sense. When we look at the numbers in the pages ahead it is curious to me the extent of the reaction compared to the crisis at hand. It appears that weather opportunistically or orchestrated we find ourselves in unprecedented times which will certainly make history.

APPENDIX C

Researchers for years have differed over the exact definition of a pandemic. The difference between an epidemic and a pandemic. Most will agree that the word describes the widespread occurrence of disease, in excess of what might normally be expected in a geographical region.

Cholera, bubonic plague, smallpox, and influenza are some of the most brutal killers in human history. And outbreaks of these diseases across international borders, are properly defined as pandemic, especially smallpox, which throughout history, has killed between 300-500 million people in its 12,000 year existence.

Originating in India the Cholera Pandemic killed over 800,000, before spreading to the Middle East, North Africa, Eastern Europe and Russia. The Sixth Cholera Pandemic was also the source of the last American outbreak of Cholera (1910–1911). American health authorities, having learned from the past, quickly sought to isolate the infected, and in the end only 11 deaths occurred in the U.S. By 1923 Cholera cases had been cut down dramatically, although it was still a constant in India.

Ravaging Europe, Africa and Asia from 1346 to 1353 the Bubonic Plague had an estimated death toll between 75 and 200 million people. Thought to have originated in Asia, the Plague most likely jumped continents via the fleas living on the rats that so frequently lived aboard merchant ships.

Smallpox is believed to have first infected humans around the time of the earliest agricultural settlements some 12,000 years ago. In the 17th and 18th centuries small pox took the toll of roughly

400 hundred thousand annually. The worldwide death toll was staggering and continued well into the twentieth century, where mortality has been estimated at 300 to 500 million. In 1980 the WHO declared it eradicated.

Considered the deadliest pandemic of the 20th century was the 1918 influenza pandemic. It was caused by an H1N1 virus with genes of avian origin. Although there is not universal consensus regarding where the virus originated, it spread worldwide during 1918-1919. In the United States, it was first identified in military personnel in spring 1918. It is estimated that about 500 million people or one-third of the world's population became infected with this virus. The number of deaths was estimated to be at least 50 million worldwide with about 675,000 occurring in the United States.

Sometimes referred to as "the Hong Kong Flu," the 1968 flu pandemic was caused by the H3N2 strain of the Influenza A virus, a genetic offshoot of the H2N2 subtype. From the first reported case on July 13, 1968 in Hong Kong, it took only 17 days before outbreaks of the virus were reported in Singapore and Vietnam, and within three months had spread to The Philippines, India, Australia, Europe, and the United States. While the 1968 pandemic had a comparatively low mortality rate (.5%) it still resulted in the deaths of more than a million people, including 500,000 residents of Hong Kong, approximately 15% of its population at the time.

Most recent in our time, first identified in Democratic Republic of the Congo in 1976, HIV/AIDS has truly proven itself as a global pandemic, killing more than 36 million people since 1981. Currently there are between 31 and 35 million people living with HIV, the vast majority of those are in Sub-Saharan Africa, where 5% of the population is infected, roughly 21 million people. As awareness has grown, new treatments have been developed that make HIV far more manageable, and many of those infected go on to lead productive lives. Between 2005 and 2012 the annual global deaths from HIV/AIDS dropped from 2.2 million to 1.6 million.

Let's put this into perspective regarding the most recent pandemics. However, it is important to acknowledge that life is a precious thing. Statistics are helpful to keep things into perspective. If the death toll were one and that one person was your … and you fill in the blank. That one death could shatter your world. That being said, let's look at the numbers. Of the three most recent the least of which was the Hong Kong Flu which claimed over 19,000 lives per week. Compared to the CoVid-19 which has claimed as of this writing late April 2020 about 231,000 lives which is roughly 11,000 per week. That's a pretty close runner up by comparison.

According to the World Health Organization the world reached phase 5 of the pandemic scale on 30th of January 2020. On March 11th, 2020 we reached phase 6 which is with human-to-human spread of virus in at least two countries in the same geographic region and extending to at least one other country outside the region. Implementation of contingency plans for health systems at all levels.

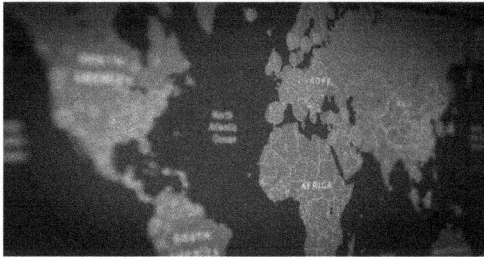

As of this writing it appears we are in the post peak stage of the pandemic.

APPENDIX D

Vitamin C Could be the Unsung COVID-19 Hero.

It appears that it's not OK in the medical community to talk about dietary supplements, like vitamin C, as a part of a treatment plan for anything, much less COVID-19. We can already see the FDA red flags are popping up. I found two recent studies by the same authors, in two separate journals about vitamin C being used to shorten the length of ICU stays and the duration of mechanical ventilation.

Even mainstream media is reporting that Long Island, New York hospitals are using vitamin C for COVID-19 patients as part of an integrative treatment. Physicians there made the decision based on experimental treatments in Wuhan, China.

"The patients who received vitamin C did significantly better than those who did not get vitamin C," said Dr. Andrew G. Weber, a pulmonologist and critical-care specialist affiliated with two Northwell Health facilities on Long Island. "It helps a tremendous amount, but it is not highlighted because it's not a sexy drug," he told the New York Post.

Two vitamin C studies authored by Harri Hemila and Elizabeth Chalker, published in *Journal of Intensive Care* and the journal *Nutrients* respectively with links to the full text.

Vitamin C may reduce the duration of mechanical ventilation in critically ill patients: a meta-regression analysis

Abstract/ Our recent meta-analysis indicated that vitamin C may shorten the length of ICU stay and the duration of mechanical ventilation. Here we analyze modification of the vitamin C effect on ventilation time, by the control group ventilation time (which we used as a proxy for severity of disease in the patients of each trial).

Methods/ The researchers searched MEDLINE, Scopus, and the Cochrane Central Register of Controlled Trials and reference lists of relevant publications. The study included controlled trials in which the administration of vitamin C was the only difference between the study groups. The research did not limit the search to randomized trials and did not require placebo control. All doses and all durations of vitamin C administration were included. One author extracted study characteristics and outcomes from the trial reports and entered the data in a spreadsheet. Both authors checked the data entered against the original reports. They used meta-regression to examine whether the vitamin C effect on ventilation time depends on the duration of ventilation in the control group.

Results/ The researchers identified nine potentially eligible trials, eight of which were included in the meta-analysis.

- They pooled the results of the eight trials, included 685 patients in total, and found that vitamin C shortened the length of mechanical ventilation on average by 14% ($P = 0.00001$).
- However, there was significant heterogeneity in the effect of vitamin C between the trials.
- Heterogeneity was fully explained by the ventilation time in the untreated control group.
- Vitamin C was most beneficial for patients with the longest ventilation, corresponding to the most severely ill patients.
- In five trials including 471 patients requiring ventilation for over 10 h, a dosage of 1-6 g/day of vitamin C shortened ventilation time on average by 25% ($P < 0.0001$).

Conclusion/ Researchers found strong evidence that vitamin C shortens the duration of mechanical ventilation, but the magnitude of the effect seems to depend on the duration of ventilation in the untreated control group. The level of baseline illness severity should be considered in further research. Different doses should be compared directly in future trials.

Vitamin C Can Shorten the Length of Stay in the ICU: A Meta-Analysis

Abstract/ A number of controlled trials have previously found that in some contexts, vitamin C can have beneficial effects on blood pressure, infections, bronchoconstriction, atrial fibrillation, and acute kidney injury. However, the practical significance of these effects is not clear. The purpose of this meta-analysis was to evaluate whether vitamin C has an effect on the practical outcomes: length of stay in the intensive care unit (ICU) and duration of mechanical ventilation.

Results/ Researchers identified 18 relevant controlled trials with a total of 2004 patients, 13 of which investigated patients undergoing elective cardiac surgery. Researchers carried out the meta-analysis using the inverse variance, fixed effect options, using the ratio of means scale.

- In 12 trials with 1766 patients, vitamin C reduced the length of ICU stay on average by 7.8% (95% CI: 4.2% to 11.2%; p = 0.00003).
- In six trials, orally administered vitamin C in doses of 1–3 g/day (weighted mean 2.0 g/day) reduced the length of ICU stay by 8.6% (p = 0.003).
- In three trials in which patients needed mechanical ventilation for over 24 hours, vitamin C shortened the duration of mechanical ventilation by 18.2% (95% CI 7.7% to 27%; p = 0.001).
- Given the insignificant cost of vitamin C, even an 8% reduction in ICU stay is worth exploring. The effects

of vitamin C on ICU patients should be investigated in more detail.

Sources: Hemilä, H., Chalker, E. Vitamin C may reduce the duration of mechanical ventilation in critically ill patients: a meta-regression analysis. *J Intensive Care*. 2020;8, 15. doi.org/10.1186/s40560-020-0432-y

Hemilä H, Chalker E. Vitamin C Can Shorten the Length of Stay in the ICU: A Meta-Analysis. *Nutrients*. 2019; 11(4):708. doi.org/10.3390/nu11040708

Online Stores:

Metagenics: http://premierhealthcare.metagenics.com/store

Practitioner Code: **PremierHealthCare**

Standard Process: https://www.standardprocess.com/Patient-Direct/patient-registration

Patient Direct Code: **WQ45V2**

RECOMMENDED READING

1. Garrett, Laurie, *The Coming Plague: Newly Emerging Diseases in a World Out of Balance*. Farrar Straus & Giroux, , (1994)

2. Appleton, Nancy,.*The Curse of Louis Pasteur*,Choice Publications (1999). Purchase from https://ifnh.org/product/the-curse-of-louis-pasteur/

3. Sompayrac, Lauren M., *How the Immune System Works*. Wiley Blackwell (2019)

4. Mathias, Christopher J. and Bannister, Sir Roger, *Autonomic Failure: A Textbook of Clinical Disorders of the Autonomic Nervous System*. Oxford University Press. (2013).

5. Wilson-Pauwels, Linda,, *Autonomic Nerves.* B.C. Decker, USA(1997).

BIBLIOGRAPHY

"The Black Death of 1348 to 1350". (2015). Retrieved from History Learning.com: https://historylearning.com/medieval-england/black-death-of-1348-to-1350/

Adams, M. (2020, February 4). *In explosive interview, author of Bioweapons Act Dr. Francis Boyle confirms coronavirus is an "offensive biological warfare weapon"*. Retrieved from Scientific News: https://scientific.news/2020-02-04-dr-francis-boyle-confirms-coronavirus-an-offensive-biological-warfare-weapon.html

Anonymous. (2020, April 3). *Why Severe Social Distancing Might Actually Result In More Coronavirus Deaths*. Retrieved from The Federalist: https://thefederalist.com/2020/04/03/why-severe-social-distancing-might-actually-result-in-more-coronavirus-deaths/

Appleton, N. (1999). The Curse of Louis Pasteur. In N. Appleton, *The Curse of Louis Pasteur*.

Bill Gates, MIT Develop New 'Tattoo ID' to Check For Vaccinations. (2019, December 23). Retrieved from 21st Century Wire.com: https://21stcenturywire.com/2019/12/23/bill-gates-develops-new-id-tattoo-to-check-for-vaccinations/

Bogumiła Kempińska-Mirosławska, A. W.-K. (2013, December 10). *The influenza epidemic of 1889–90 in selected European cities – a picture based on the reports of two Poznań daily newspapers from the second half of the nineteenth century.* Retrieved from NCBI: https://www.ncbi.nlm.nih.gov/pmc/articles/PMC3867475/citedby/

CHANG, B. C. (2020, April 20). *Miami-Dade has tens of thousands of missed coronavirus infections, UM survey finds.* Retrieved from Miami Herald: https://www.miamiherald.com/news/coronavirus/article242260406.html

Chastain, J. (2020, April 6). *FBI arrests Charles Lieber for selling the COVID-19 to China?* Retrieved from Daily US Times.com: https://www.dailyustimes.com/fbi-arrests-charles-lieber-for-selling-the-covid-19-to-china/

Christopher J. Mathias and, R. B. (2013). Autonomic Failure: A Textbook of Clinical Disorders of the Autonomic Nervous System. In R. B. Christopher J. Mathias and, *Autonomic Failure: A Textbook of Clinical Disorders of the Autonomic Nervous System.* Oxford University Press.

Cold Arrest. (1994). Retrieved from Furture World: https://future-world.com/mcatalog/

Conark, B. (2020, April 10). *News.* Retrieved from MiamiHerald.com: https://www.miamiherald.com/news/coronavirus/article241869876.html

Coronavirus disease 2019 (COVID-19). (2020, March 6). Retrieved from World Health Organization: https://www.who.int/docs/default-source/coronaviruse/situation-reports/20200306-sitrep-46-covid-19.pdf?sfvrsn=96b04adf_2

COVID-19 Resource Centre. (2020). Retrieved from The Lancet: https://www.thelancet.com/ coronavirus?dgcid=kr_pop-up_tlcoronavirus20

David Perlin, P. a. (2002). *Epidemics of the Past: Smallpox.* Retrieved from Infoplease: https://www. infoplease.com/math-science/health/diseases/ epidemics-of-the-past-smallpox-12000-years-of-terror

Dr. Liji Thomas, M. (2020, March 31). *Eight strains of coronavirus afflicting the world.* Retrieved from News Medical Life Sciences: https://www.news-medical.net/news/20200331/ Eight-strains-of-coronavirus-afflicting-the-world.aspx

Dresden, D. (2020, March 12). *Coronavirus vaccine: Everything you need to know.* Retrieved from Medical News Today: https://www.medicalnewstoday.com/articles/ coronavirus-vaccine

Engineering, J. H. (2020). *TODAY'S CORONAVIRUS TRACKER.* Retrieved from Associations Now: https:// associationsnow.com/coronavirus-tracker/

Florida Covid-19 Response. (2020). Retrieved from Florida Health: https://floridahealthcovid19.gov/

Garrett, L. (1994). The Coming Plague: Newly Emerging Diseases in a World Out of Balance. In L. Garrett, *The Coming Plague: Newly Emerging Diseases in a World Out of Balance.* Macmillan.

Golding, L. M. (2020, March 24). *New York hospitals treating coronavirus patients with vitamin C.* Retrieved from New York Post: https://nypost.com/2020/03/24/new-york- hospitals-treating-coronavirus-patients-with-vitamin-c/

Grice EA1, S. J. (2011, August). *The skin microbiome.* Retrieved from Pub Med: https://www.ncbi.nlm.nih.gov/pubmed/21407241

Group, U. M. (2020). *HOW MANY PEOPLE DIE FROM THE FLU EVERY YEAR IN THE US?* Retrieved from Urgent Medical Center: http://www.urgentcarefl.com/many-people-die-flu-every-year-us/

Halaschak, Z. (2020, March 28). *'Immortal' Italian woman, 102, survives coronavirus infection.* Retrieved from The Washington Examiner: https://www.washingtonexaminer.com/news/immortal-italian-woman-102-survives-coronavirus-infection

Hemilä, H. (2019, March 27). *Vitamin C Can Shorten the Length of Stay in the ICU: A Meta-Analysis.* Retrieved from Nutrients 2019: https://www.mdpi.com/2072-6643/11/4/708

Hemilä, H. C. (2020). *Vitamin C may reduce the duration of mechanical ventilation in critically ill patients.* Retrieved from Journal of Intensive Care volume 8, Article number15: https://jintensivecare.biomedcentral.com/articles/10.1186/s40560-020-0432-y#citeas

Hopper, L. (2020, April 20). *Early antibody testing suggests COVID-19 infections in L.A. County greatly exceed documented cases.* Retrieved from USC News: https://news.usc.edu/168987/antibody-testing-results-covid-19-infections-los-angeles-county/

J Rocklöv, P. H.-S. (2020, February 28). *COVID-19 outbreak on the Diamond Princess cruise ship: estimating the epidemic potential and effectiveness of public health countermeasures.* Retrieved from Journal of Travel Medicine: https://academic.oup.com/jtm/advance-article/doi/10.1093/jtm/taaa030/5766334

Kahn, J. S., & McIntosh, K. M. (2005, November-Volume 24 - Issue 11 - p S223-S227). *History and Recent Advances in Coronavirus Discovery*. Retrieved from The Pediatric Infectious Disease Journal: https://journals.lww.com/pidj/pages/articleviewer.aspx?year=2005&issue=11001&article=00012&type=Fulltext

Koenig, D. (2020, April 17). *How Accurate Are Coronavirus Death Counts?* Retrieved from WebMD.com: https://www.webmd.com/lung/news/20200417/how-accurate-are-coronavirus-death-counts

Lab, H. G. (2020). *Novel Coronavirus Infection Map*. Retrieved from University of Washington: https://hgis.uw.edu/virus/

LINDA WILSON-PAUWELS, P. A. (1997). Autonomic Nerves . In P. A. LINDA WILSON-PAUWELS, *Autonomic Nerves* . PMPH, USA.

Lyons-Weiler, J. (2020, April 3). *Is CDC Borrowing Pneumonia Deaths "From Flu" for "From COVID-19?* Retrieved from LinkedIn: https://www.linkedin.com/pulse/cdc-borrowing-pneumonia-deaths-from-flu-covid-19-james-lyons-weiler

McDermott-Murphy, C. (2020, February 14). *The Harvard Gazette*. Retrieved from https://news.harvard.edu/gazette/story/2020/02/how-crispr-technology-is-advancing/

Mike Adams. (2014, October 19). *ALERT: U.S. Army researchers at USAMRIID confirm Ebola variant was airborne in 1990*. Retrieved from Natural News.com: https://www.naturalnews.com/047317_Ebola_Reston_airborne_transmission_USAMRIID.html

Mills-Gregg, D. (2020, January 6). *US Military Bases Ramp Up Security Measures Amid Threats from Iran.* Retrieved from Military.com: https://www.military.com/daily-news/2020/01/06/us-bases-ramp-security-measures-amid-threats-iran.html

Moriarty LF, P. M. (2020, March 23). *Public Health Responses to COVID-19 Outbreaks on Cruise Ships-Worldwide.* Retrieved from Center for Disease Control: https://www.cdc.gov/mmwr/volumes/69/wr/mm6912e3.htm#suggestedcitation

Neil M Ferguson, D. L.-G. (2020, March 16). *Report 9: Impact of non-pharmaceutical interventions (NPIs) to reduce COVID-19 mortality and healthcare demand.* Retrieved from Imperial College London: https://www.imperial.ac.uk/media/imperial-college/medicine/mrc-gida/2020-03-16-COVID19-Report-9.pdf

O'Neil, C. (2020, April 13). *10 Reasons to Doubt the Covid-19 Data.* Retrieved from Bloomberg: https://www.bloomberg.com/opinion/articles/2020-04-13/ten-reasons-to-doubt-the-covid-19-data

panelYueWangaYiZhangbYan-qinShiaXian-huaPanaYan-huaLubPingCaoc, A. l. (2018, March). *Antibacterial effects of cinnamon (Cinnamomum zeylanicum) bark essential oil on Porphyromonas gingivalis.* Retrieved from Science Direct: https://www.sciencedirect.com/science/article/abs/pii/S0882401017313918

PYGAS, M. (2014, June 30). *10 Amazing Female Spies Who Brought Down The Nazis.* Retrieved from ListVerse.com: https://listverse.com/2013/09/05/10-women-spies-who-brought-down-the-third-reich/

Richardson, V. (2020, April 20). *USC antibody study shows coronavirus 'far more widespread,' death rate 'much lower'*. Retrieved from The Washington Times: https://www.washingtontimes.com/news/2020/apr/20/coronavirus-antibody-study-shows-covid-19-far-more/

Roujian Lu, X. Z. (2020, February 22). *The Lancet*. Retrieved from https://www.thelancet.com/journals/lancet/article/PIIS0140-6736(20)30251-8/fulltext

Seidel, J. (2020, January 29). Retrieved from News.com.au: https://www.news.com.au/lifestyle/health/health-problems/mystery-lab-next-to-coronavirus-epicentre/news-story/3e5a32fe77263fe8ca81b091cc8d9c42

Shilhavy, B. (2015, February 17). *"Mass Sterilization": Kenyan Doctors Find Anti-fertility Agent in UN Tetanus Vaccine*. Retrieved from Global Reasearch: https://www.globalresearch.ca/mass-sterilization-kenyan-doctors-find-anti-fertility-agent-in-un-tetanus-vaccine/5431664

Sompayrac, L. M. (2012). How the Immune System Works. In L. M. Sompayrac, *How the Immune System Works*. Wiley Blackwell .

Stanford Study Indicates COVID-19 Cases Far More Widespread Than Reported. (2020, April 18). Retrieved from MSN.com: https://www.msn.com/en-us/news/us/stanford-study-indicates-covid-19-cases-far-more-widespread-than-reported/ar-B

Vogel, L. (2011, September 6). *Hand sanitizers may increase norovirus risk*. Retrieved from NCBI: https://www.ncbi.nlm.nih.gov/pmc/articles/PMC3168661/citedby/

Wade, N. (2010, October 31). *Europe's Plagues Came From China, Study Finds.* Retrieved from New Yourk Times.com: https://www.nytimes.com/2010/11/01/health/01plague.html?_r=0

ACKNOWLEDGEMENTS

I want to recognize and offer my thanks to the following people for helping me publish this book:

For the hours of guidance and editing along with the encouragement to transform my initial stacks of research into a published piece to help and guide others, I thank Leonard Szymczak a fellow Toastmaster, mentor, and friend.

The patients, family and friends who read through the first draft and offered valuable feedback on the material and how it came across I owe much gratitude and thanks. Including Carole Cochrane, Susan Taylor, Anthony Gioutsos, Britany Doyle, Ted Haun, Tom Gertsen, and Lisette Campbell. Also, the many patients along with those in my Toastmasters group who I shared some of the content with to help refine it in a way that is more helpful. Those who endured undoubtedly more explanation of technical material than was expected. Thank you.

Also, a friend and resource of tremendous information Ted Haun who assisted in the protocols with me as well as helping with research, I am indebted.

I greatly appreciate Lauren Card for her patience and creative expertise in the cover design as well as the many revisions and changes along the way. For helping with pictures and table formatting as well as a sounding board for ideas.

Thanks to Tamara Cribley for her efforts and expertise with interior design and layout of the book. I appreciate her expertise and patience with the process which was certainly a learning experience for me.

Thank you to Kathryn Brunk and her meticulous keen eye in punctuation, spelling, and grammar correction.

There may be someone, or several some ones I did not mention, those that sparked an idea or shared insight as things developed. Many thanks and gratitude for being part of the process.

ABOUT THE AUTHOR

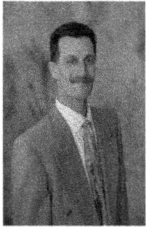

Dr. Bradley Shapero, D.C. is a wellness doctor and chiropractor, has been serving the communities of South Orange County for over 28 years in the field of Wellness, Chiropractic and Therapeutic Lifestyle Changes. Dr. Shapero grew up in Southern California and acquired his degree from Cleveland Chiropractic College of Los Angles.

He is active in the community and specializes in all aspects of Family Health Care with an emphasis on children and anti-aging. Dr. Shapero contributes and participates in various programs such as Character Counts through the Orange County Sheriffs Dept., Local Chambers of Commerce, Community Food Drives, and Toys for Tots and many others.

Having a passion to help people and a talent for solving difficult and chronic cases, Dr. Shapero deals with Headaches, Arthritis, Fibromyalgia, ADD, Chronic Fatigue, Back Pain, Digestive Disorders such as irritable bowl and diverticulitis, Allergies, hormone imbalances, Sports injuries, and many more.

Outside his busy practice Dr. Shapero also volunteers for the Foundations of Wellness Professionals for which he presents regular educational workshops to the community on various topics that he specializes in; including Anti-aging, Balancing Hormones Naturally, Five Secrets to Permanent Weight Loss, The Three Solutions to Health, Corporate Wellness, Restoring Your Mojo, ADHD as well as many others.

His intention is to give up-to-date information to create a healthier tomorrow.

For more information, visit his websites:

www.PremierHealthCareSC.com
www.DrBradShaperoOnline.com

Dr. Shapero may be contacted at
DrShapero@PremierHealthCareSC.com

www.ingramcontent.com/pod-product-compliance
Lightning Source LLC
Chambersburg PA
CBHW052205270326
41931CB00011B/2236